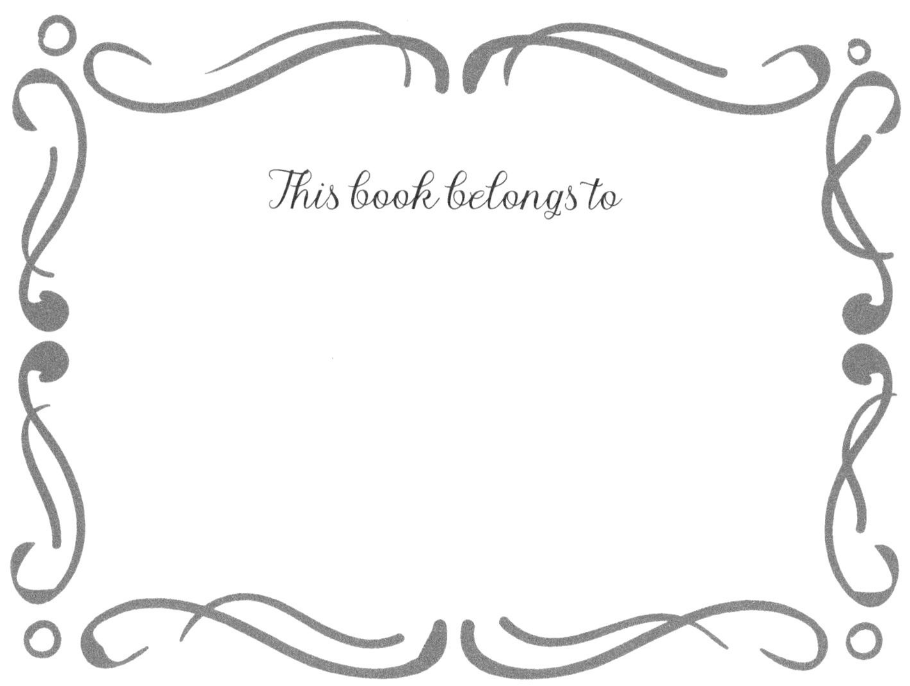

This book belongs to

Game Rules

for couple

Take turns and choose between
TRUTH or **DARE**.

If you don't answer the truth question or complete
your dare, your partner can choose your "punishment".

P.s. You are only allowed 5 truths!

Game Rules

Every player sits in a circle, then an empty bottle is placed on a table or on the ground.

- Palyer 1 begins by rotating the bottle.

   The bottleneck now points to player 2.

- Player 2 choose **TRUTH** or **DARE**

   If a dare is chosen, player 2 turns the bottle again to find his/her dare partner!

If player 2 does not answer the truth question or complete his/her dare, player 1 can choose his/her "punishment"!

P.s. Each player are only allowed 5 truths!

#1
TRUTH

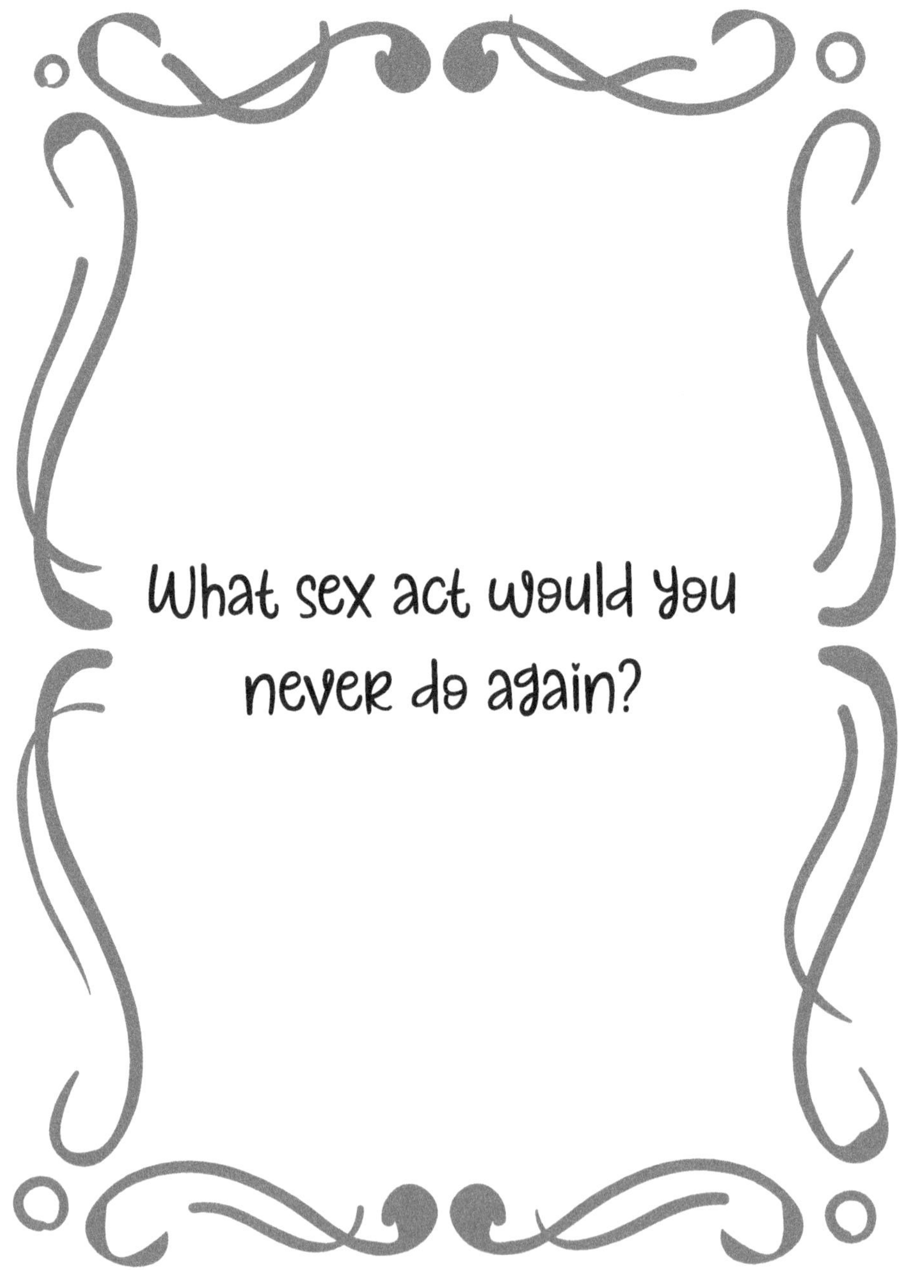

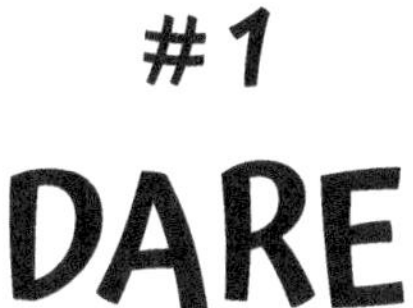

#1
DARE

Close your eyes, scroll through your contacts list and tell me the sexiest thing about the person you land on.

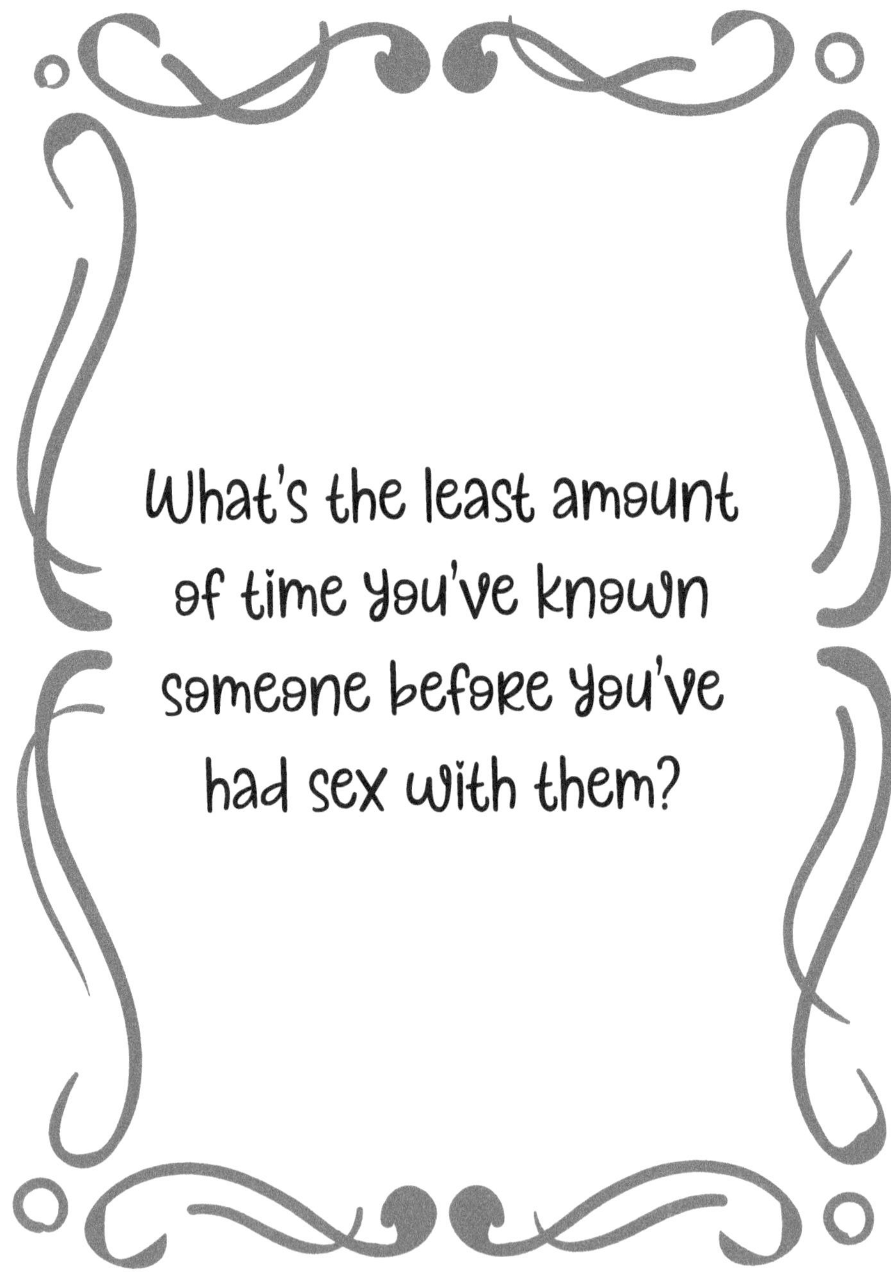

2

TRUTH

What's the least amount
of time you've known
someone before you've
had sex with them?

#2
DARE

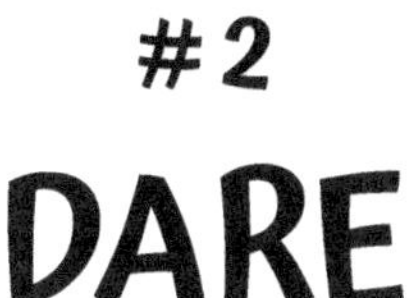

Sing the chorus of a song
you've had sex to.

DARE

#3
TRUTH

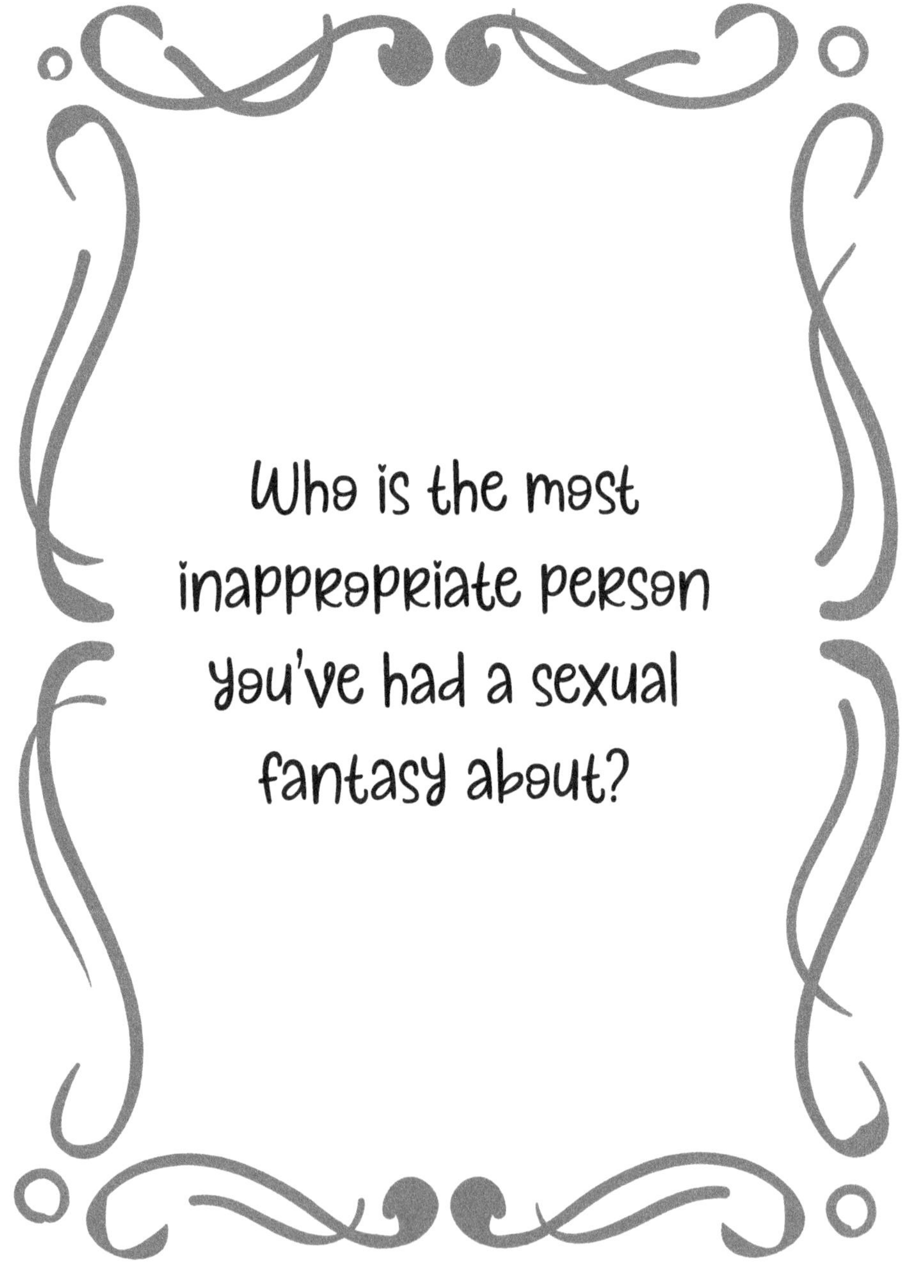

Who is the most inappropriate person you've had a sexual fantasy about?

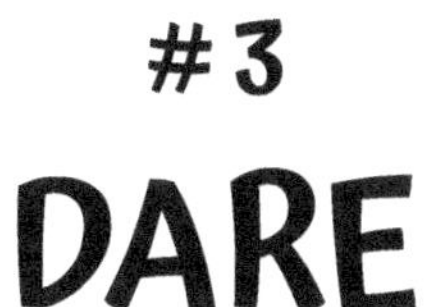

3
DARE

Suck on my finger and pretend you're performing oral sex for 30 seconds.

DARE

#4
TRUTH

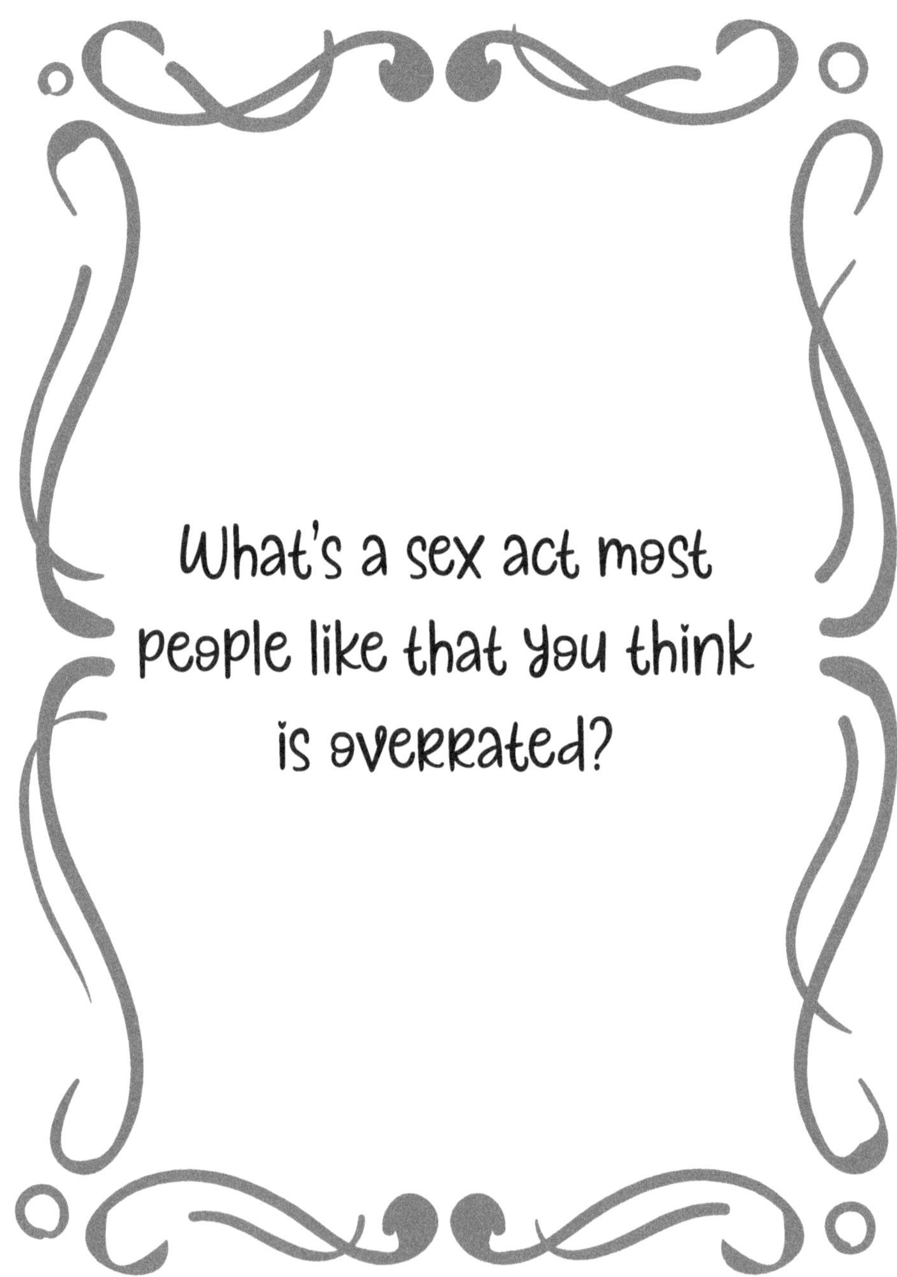

What's a sex act most people like that you think is overrated?

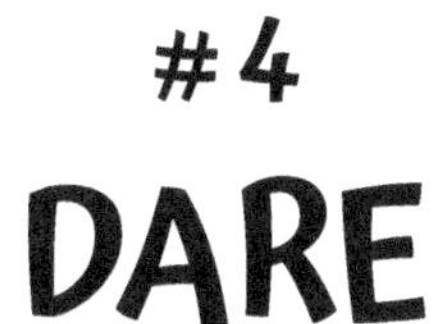

#4
DARE

Call a local pizza place and try to convince someone that you need a "special" delivery person.

DARE

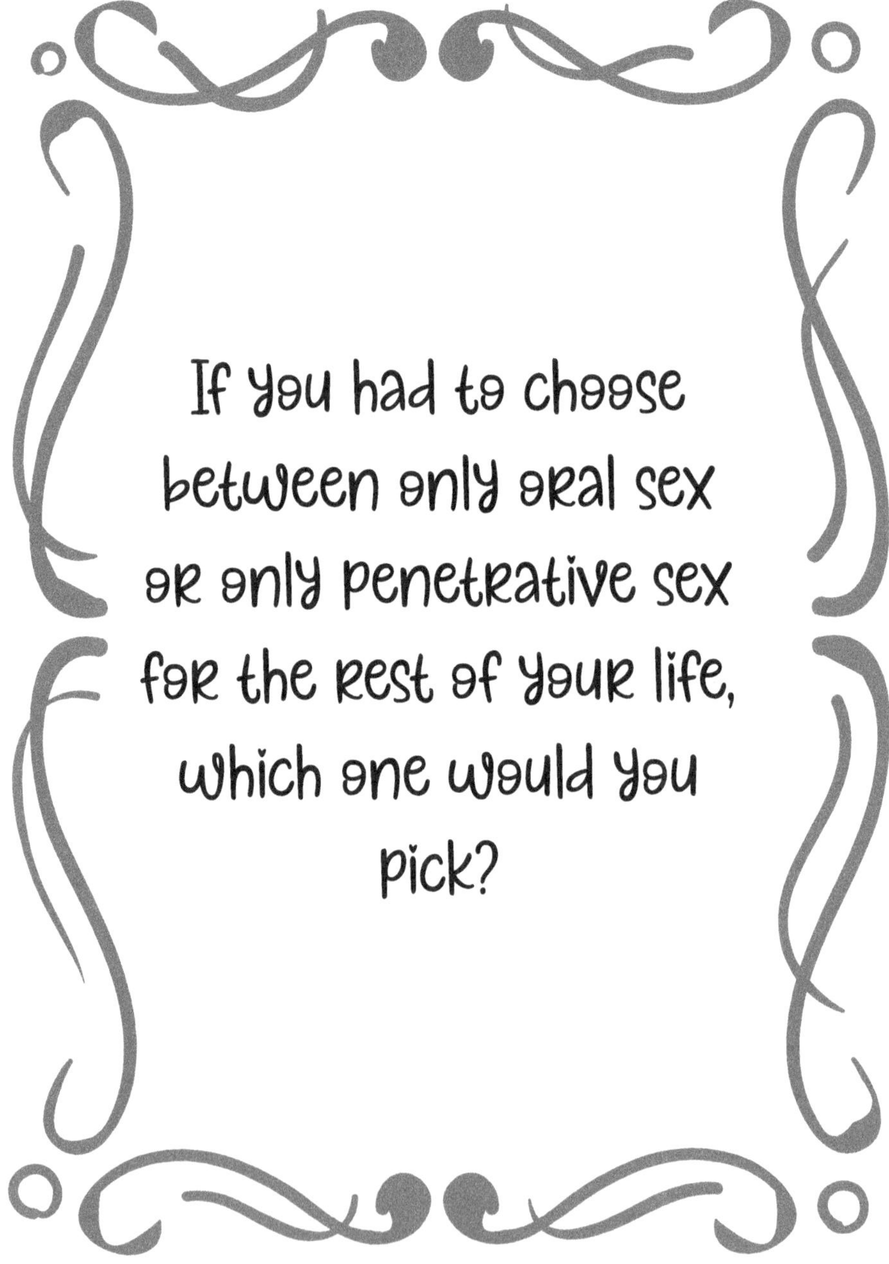

#5
TRUTH

If you had to choose between only oral sex or only penetrative sex for the rest of your life, which one would you pick?

#5
DARE

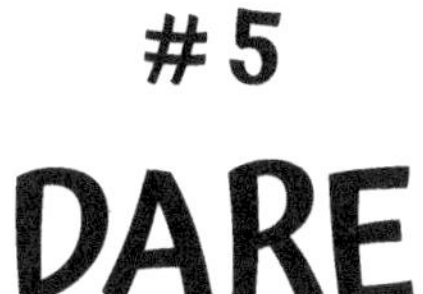

Send a suggestive text
message to someone in
your phone.

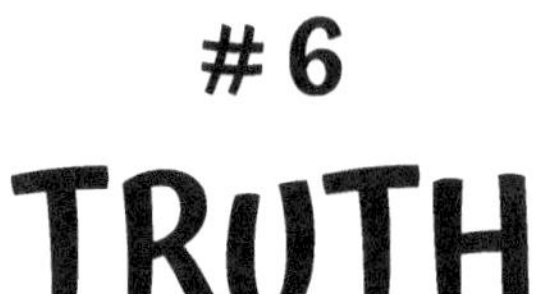

#6
TRUTH

Is sex better when you're in love, or better when the other person is hot and mysterious?

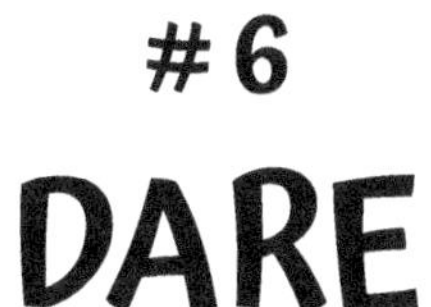

Put a blindfold on and kiss
whatever body part I put
in front of your mouth.

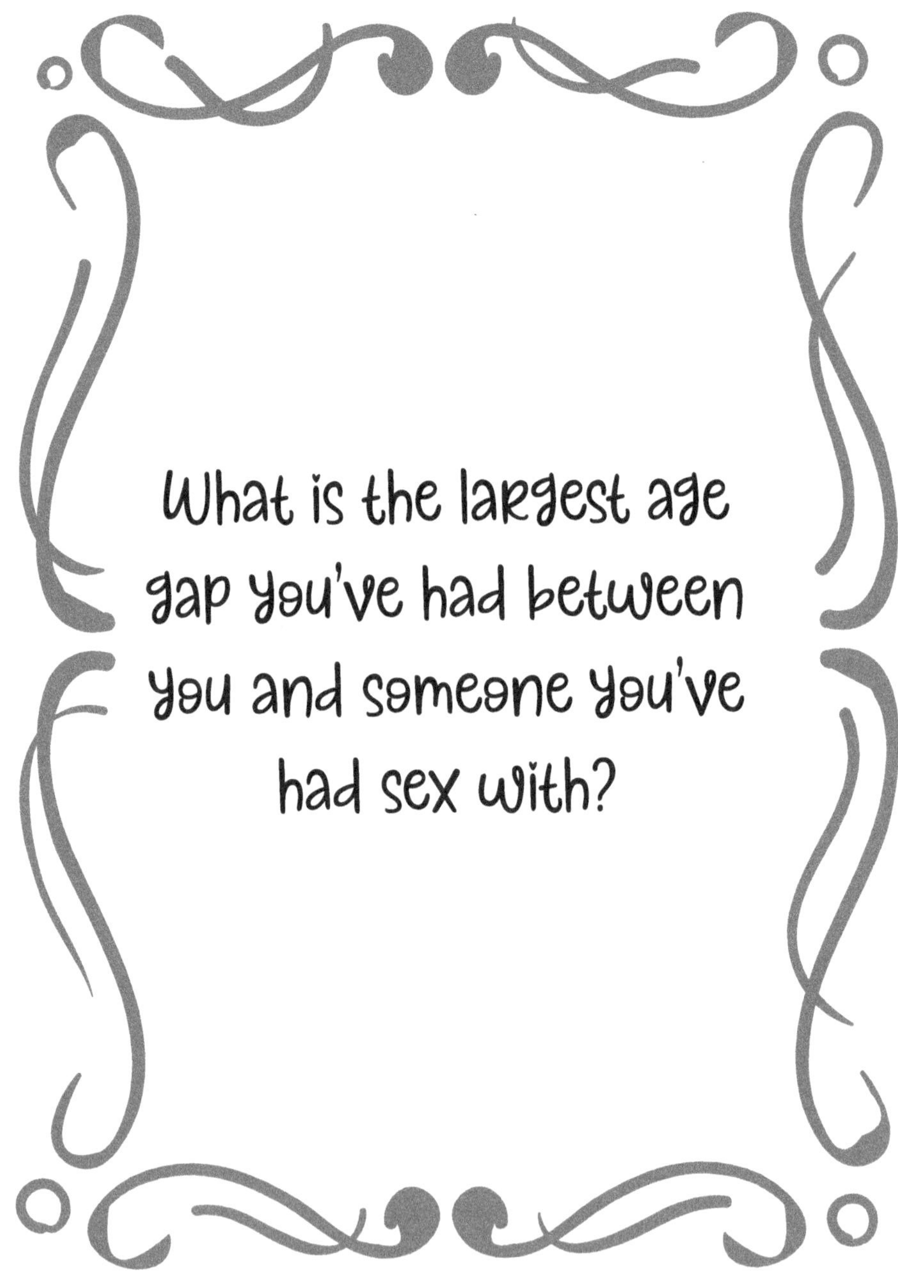

#7
TRUTH

What is the largest age gap you've had between you and someone you've had sex with?

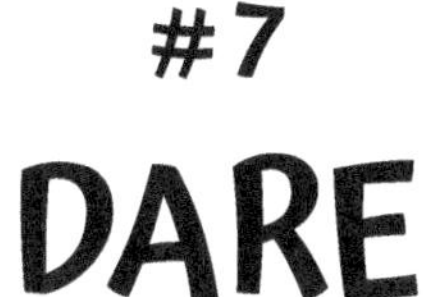

#7
DARE

Let me lick your lips and you have to resist kissing or touching me the whole time.

#8
TRUTH

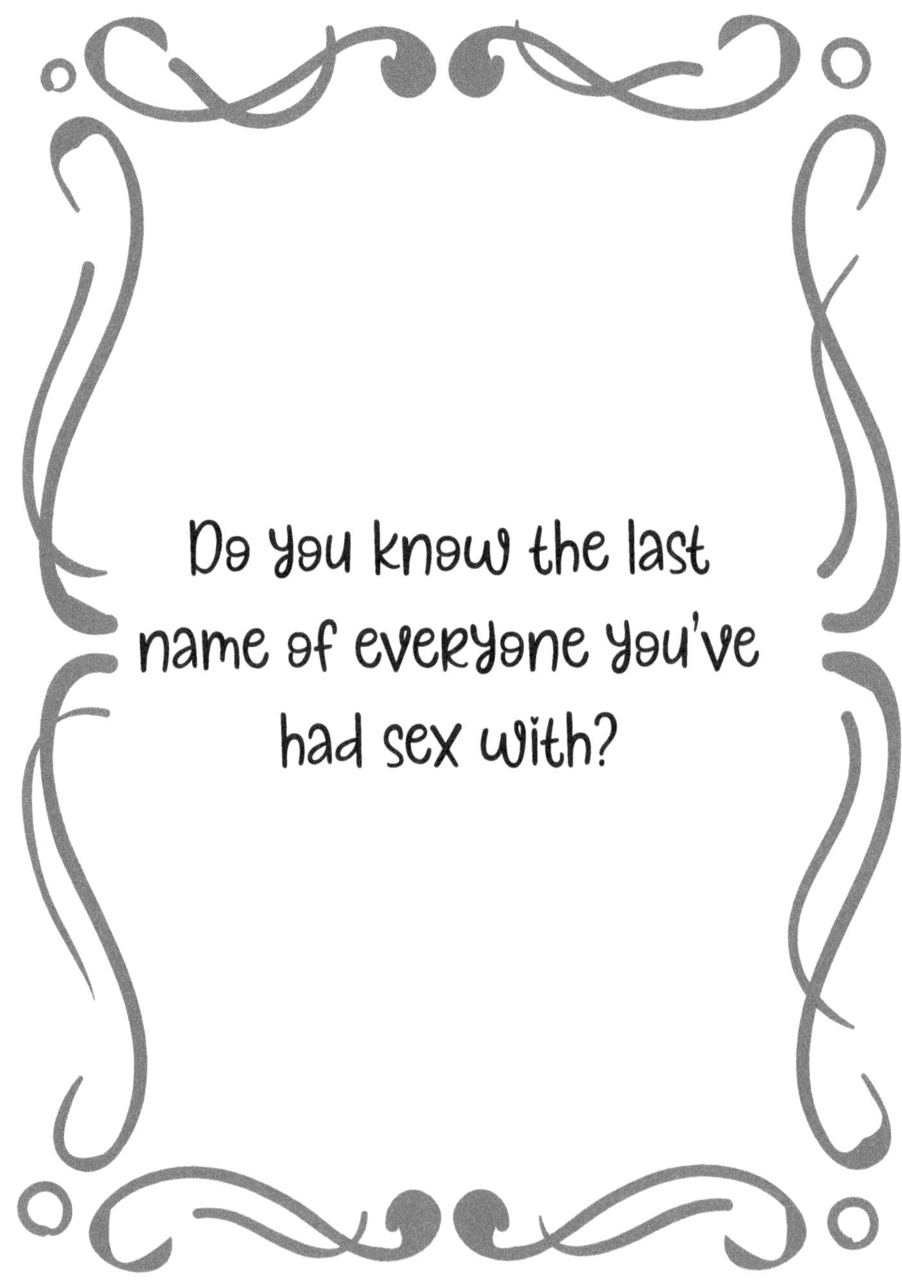

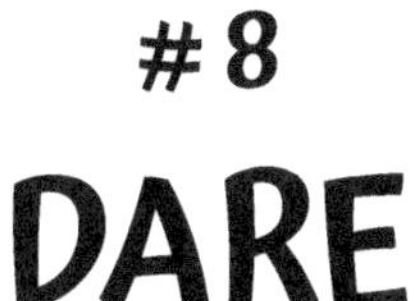

#8
DARE

Put something edible on my forearm and lick it off.

#9
TRUTH

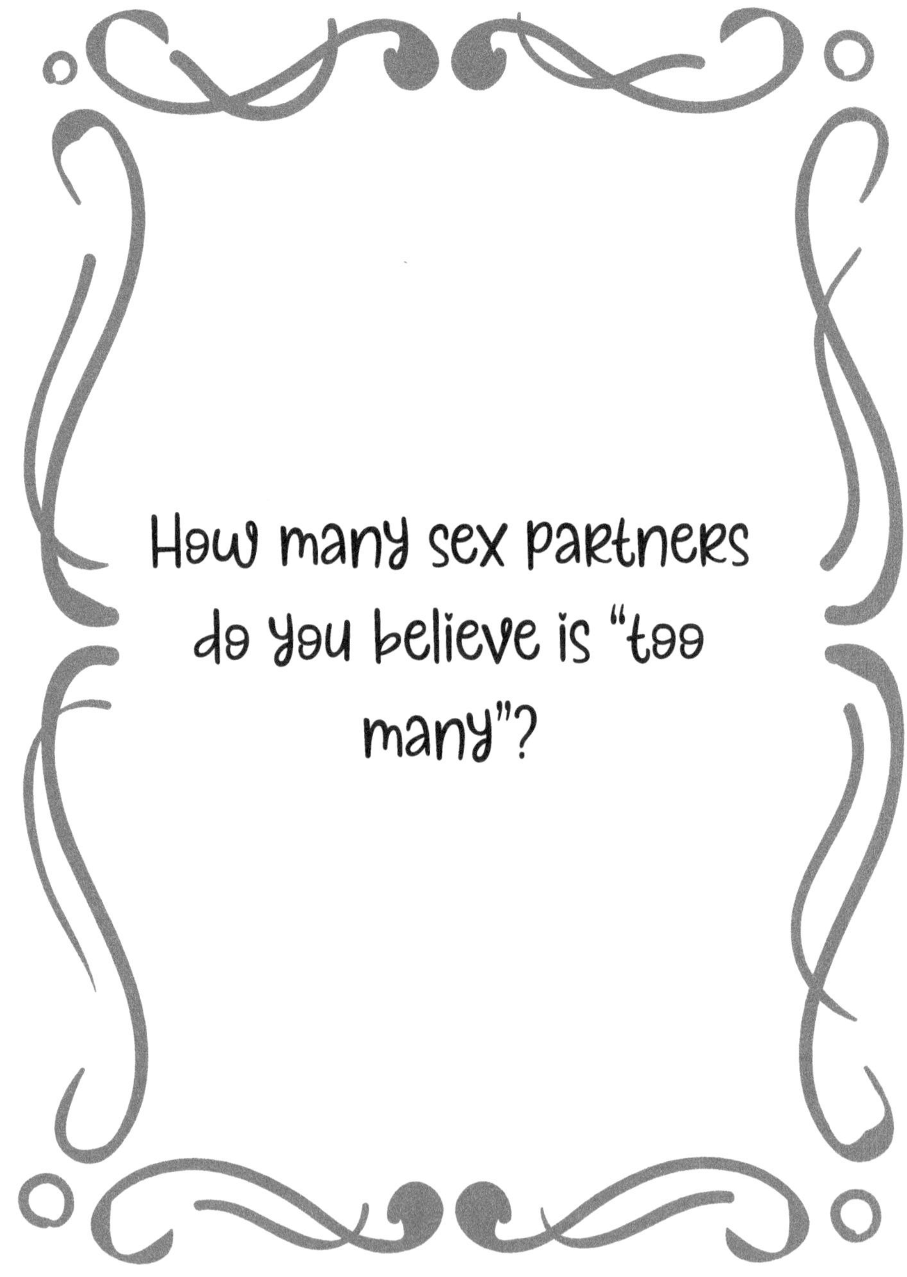

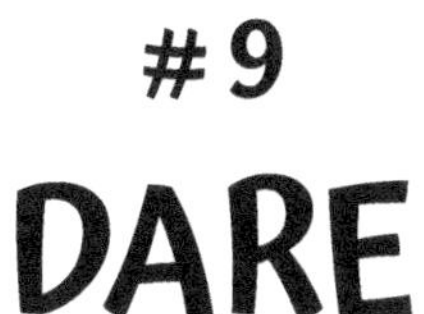

#9
DARE

Go in the bathroom and take a suggestive selfie and send it to me.

#10
TRUTH

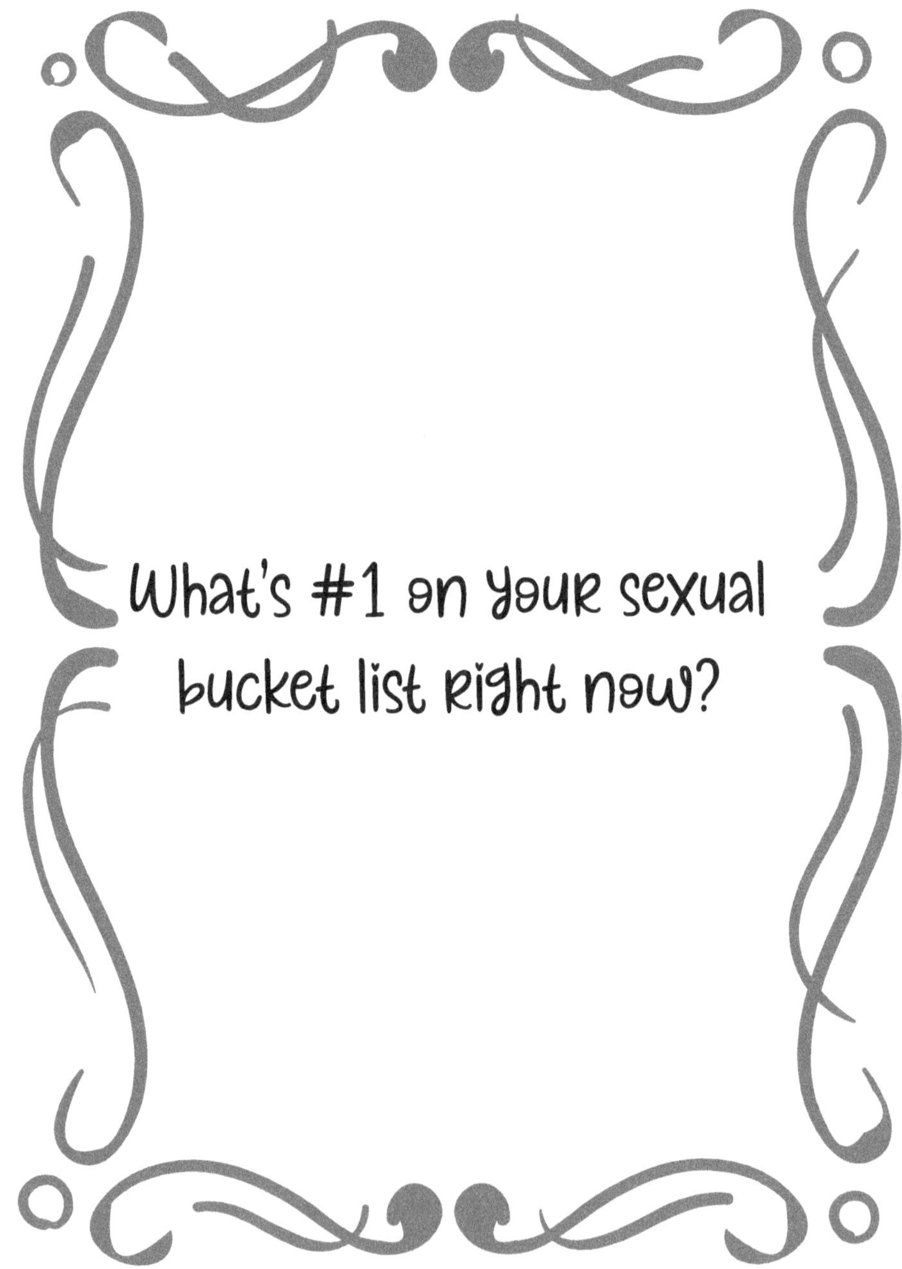

What's #1 on your sexual
bucket list right now?

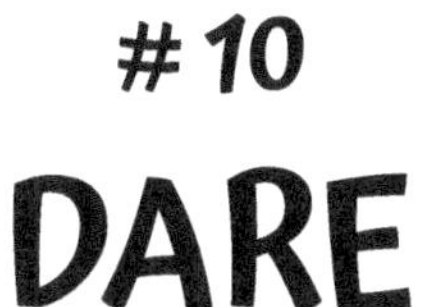

#10
DARE

Send a Facebook message to someone you've slept with describing a dirty dream you've had about them.

#11
TRUTH

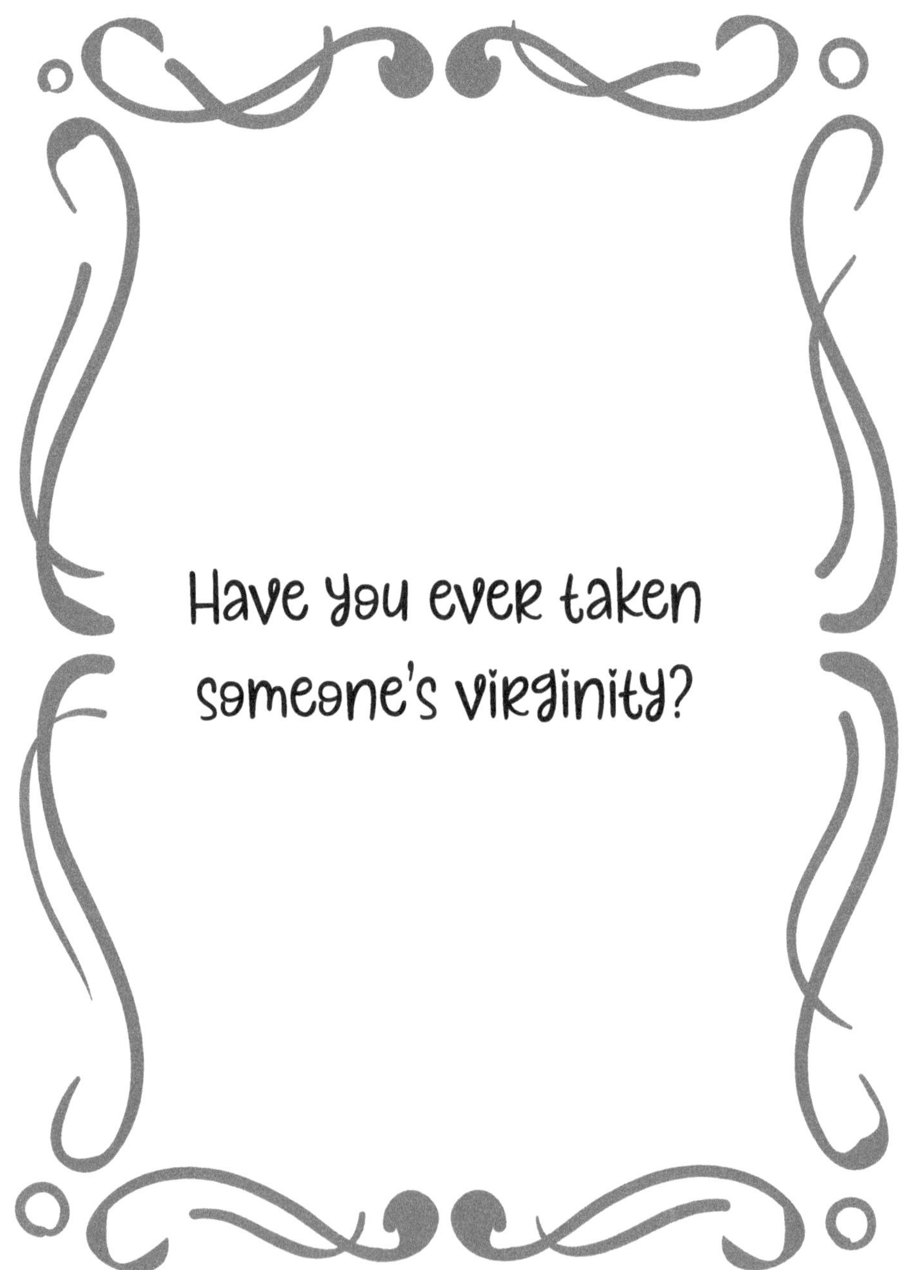

Have you ever taken
someone's virginity?

#11
DARE

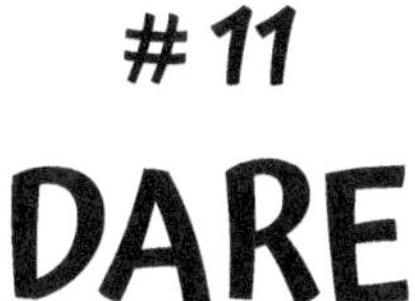

Call a phone sex line and pretend that you have a diaper fetish.

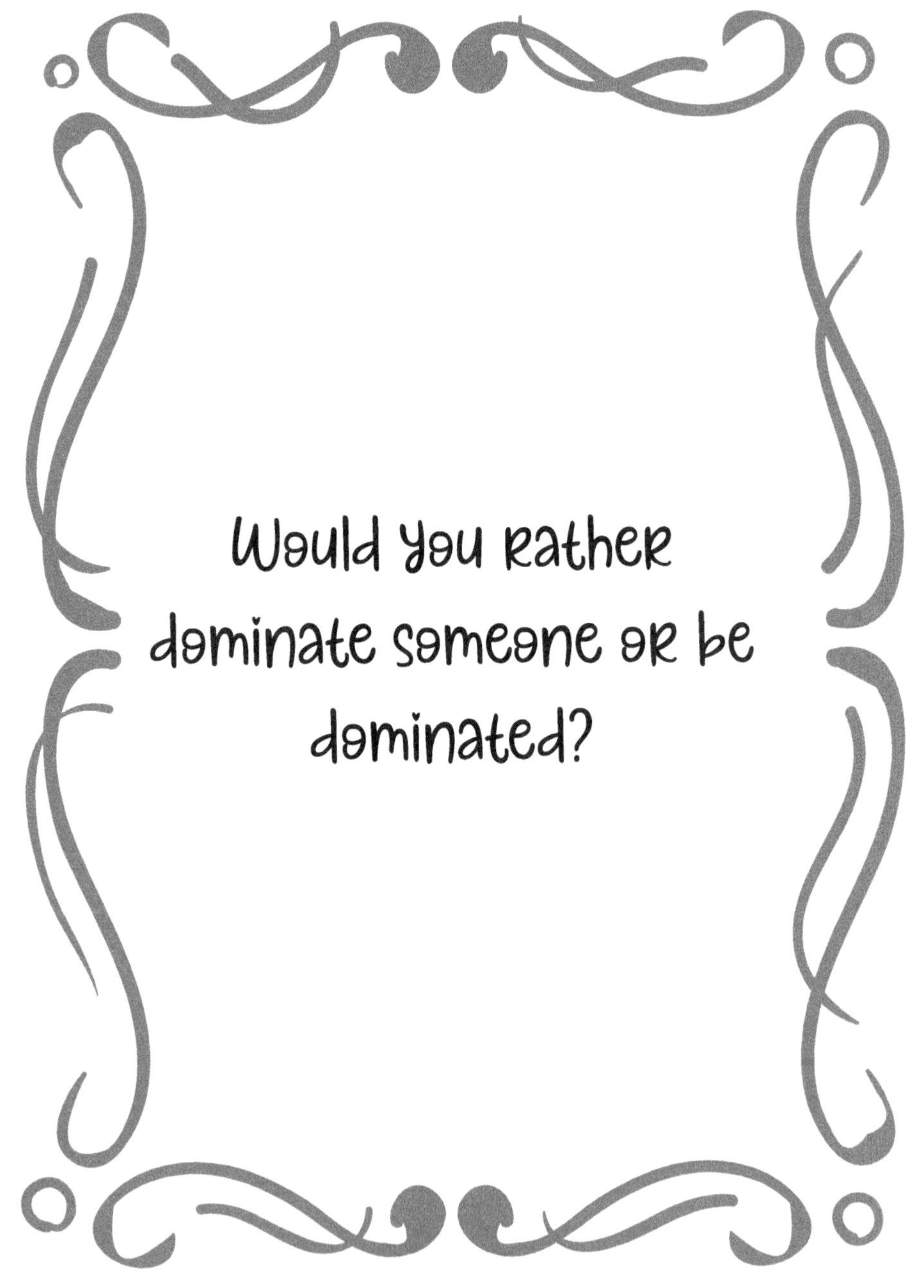

12
TRUTH

Would you rather dominate someone or be dominated?

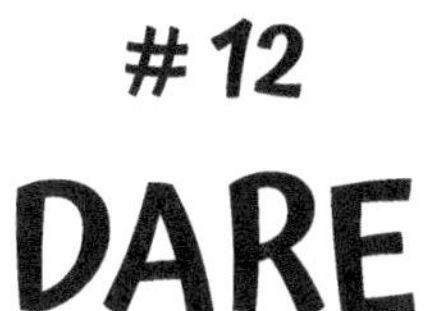

DARE

Put a blindfold on and try
to guess which body part
I'm touching you with.

#13
TRUTH

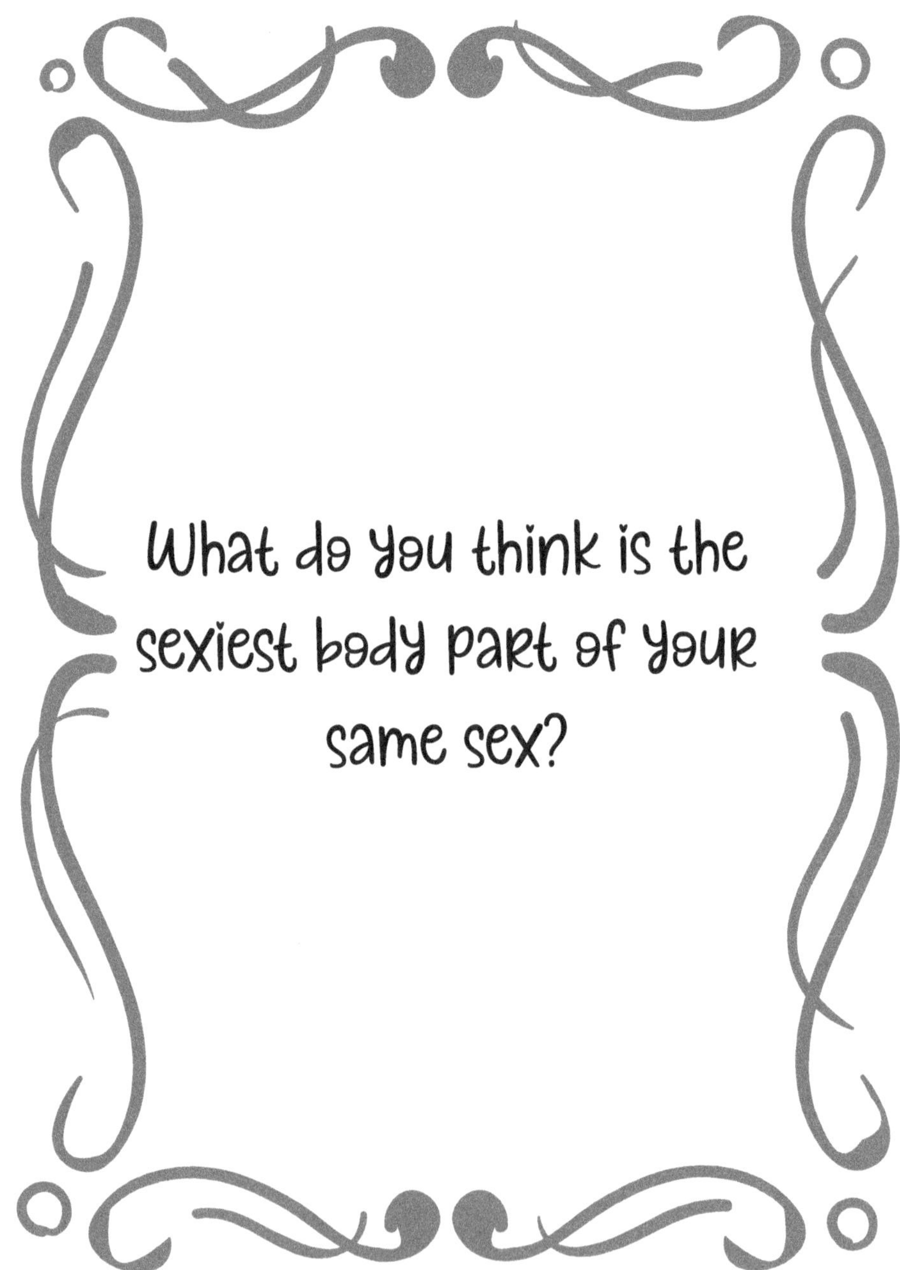

What do you think is the sexiest body part of your same sex?

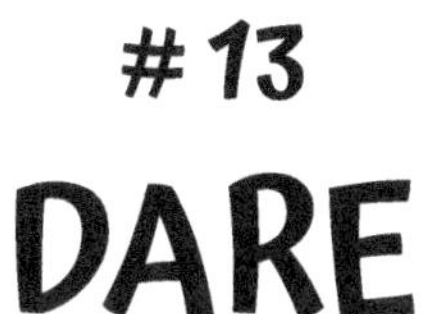

#13
DARE

Whisper something in my ear that you think will turn me on.

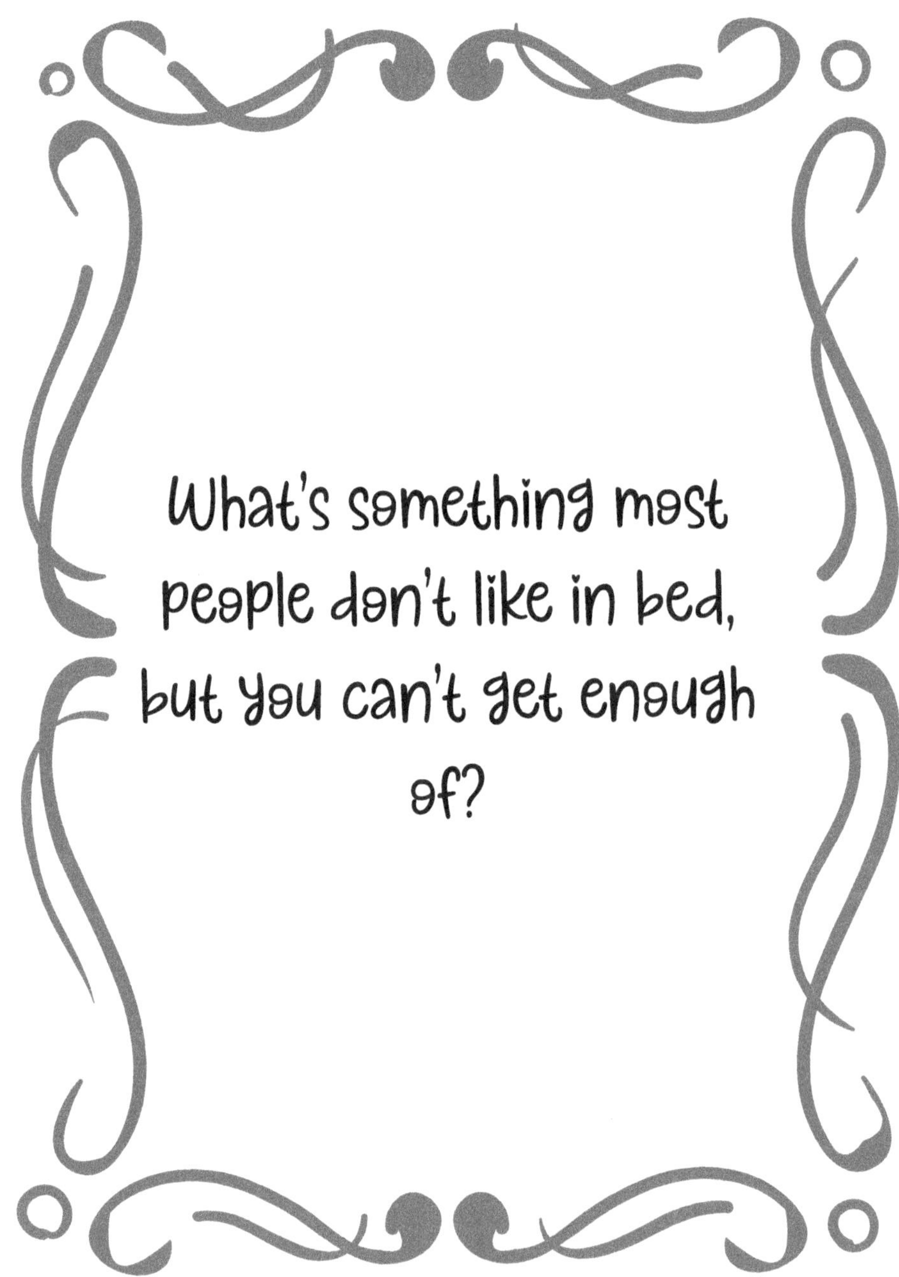

#14
TRUTH

What's something most people don't like in bed, but you can't get enough of?

#14
DARE

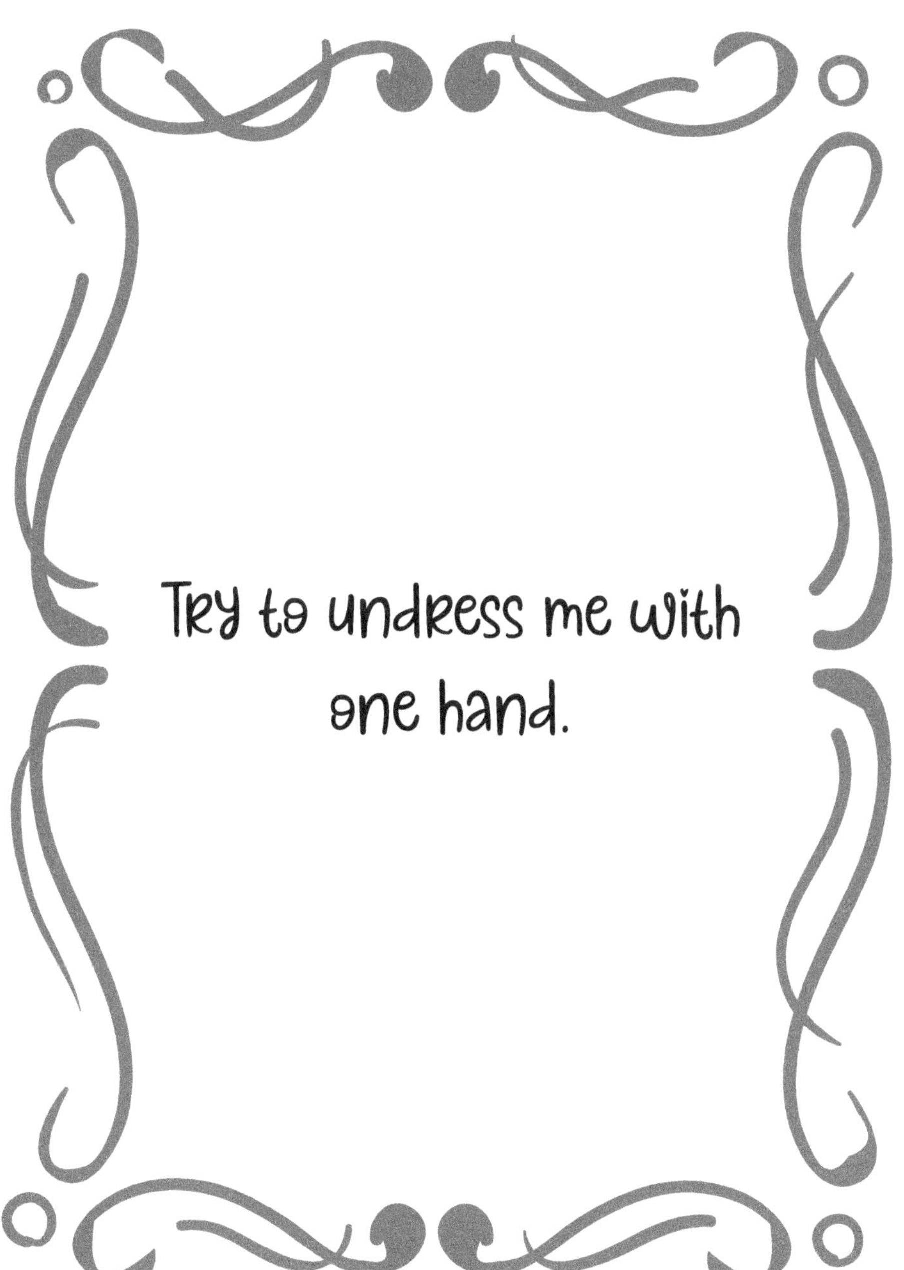

Try to undress me with
one hand.

15
TRUTH

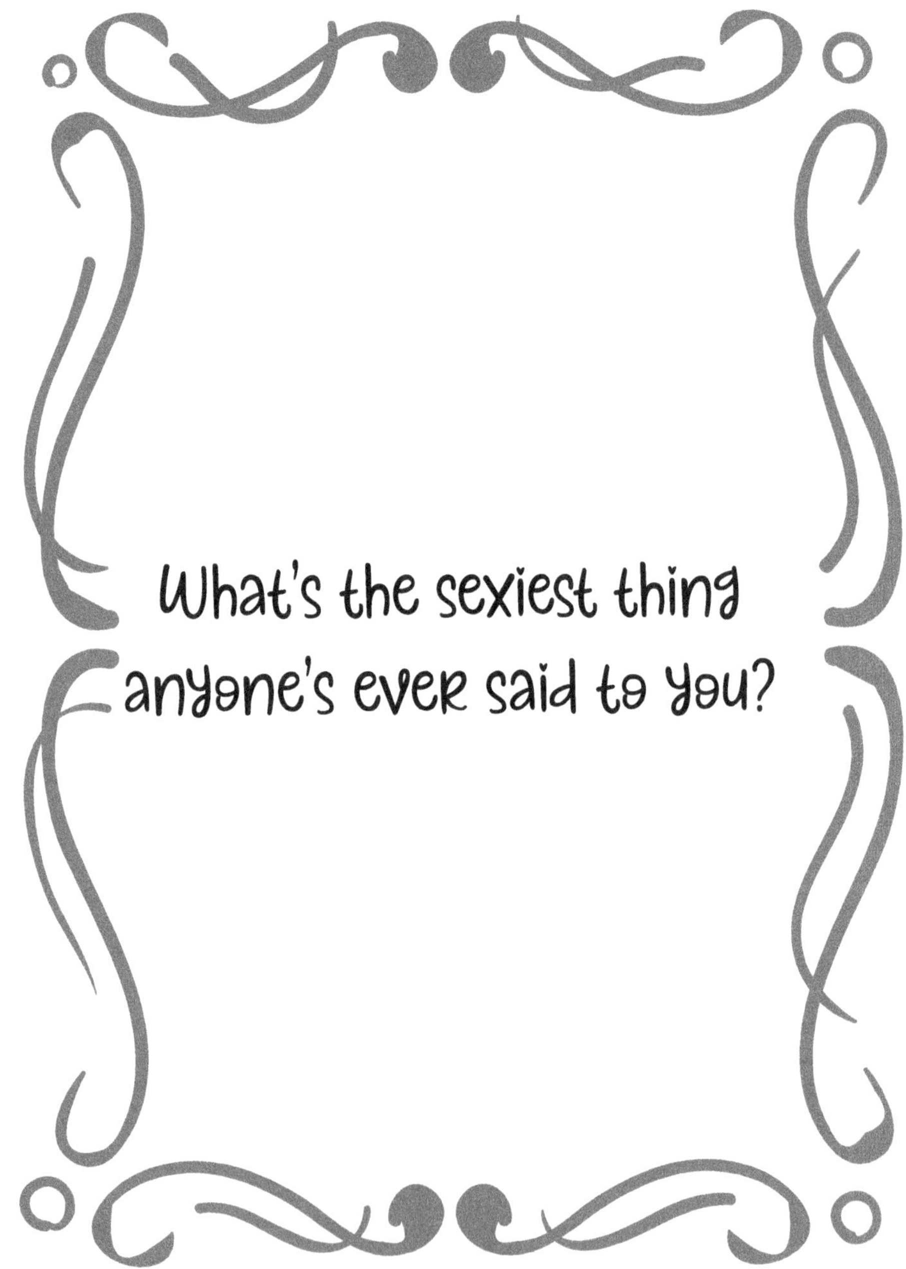

What's the sexiest thing
anyone's ever said to you?

#15
DARE

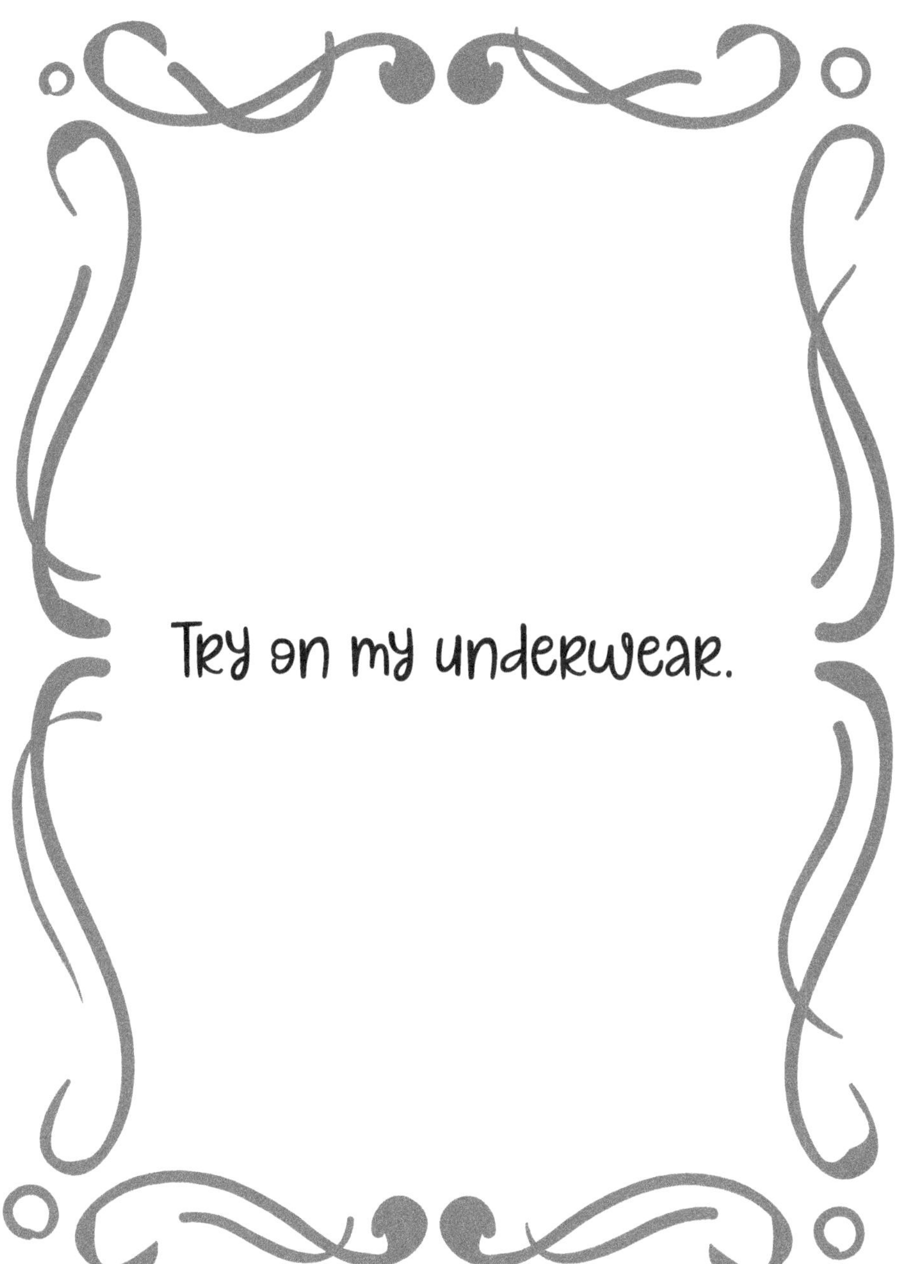

16
TRUTH

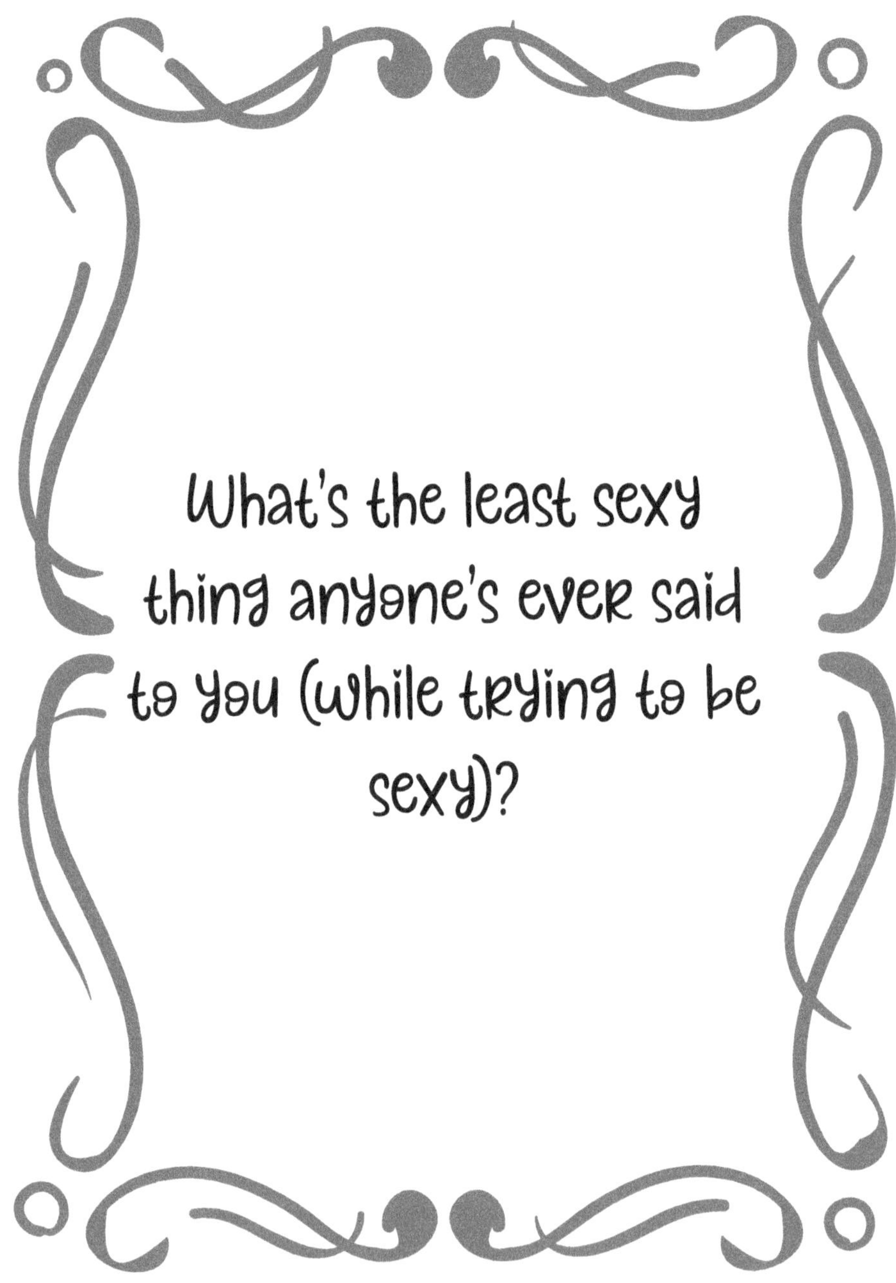

What's the least sexy thing anyone's ever said to you (while trying to be sexy)?

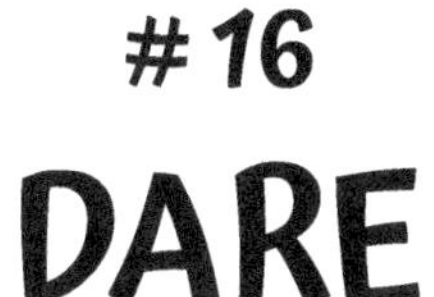

#16
DARE

Use one of your sex toys on yourself for 60 seconds.

DARE

#17
TRUTH

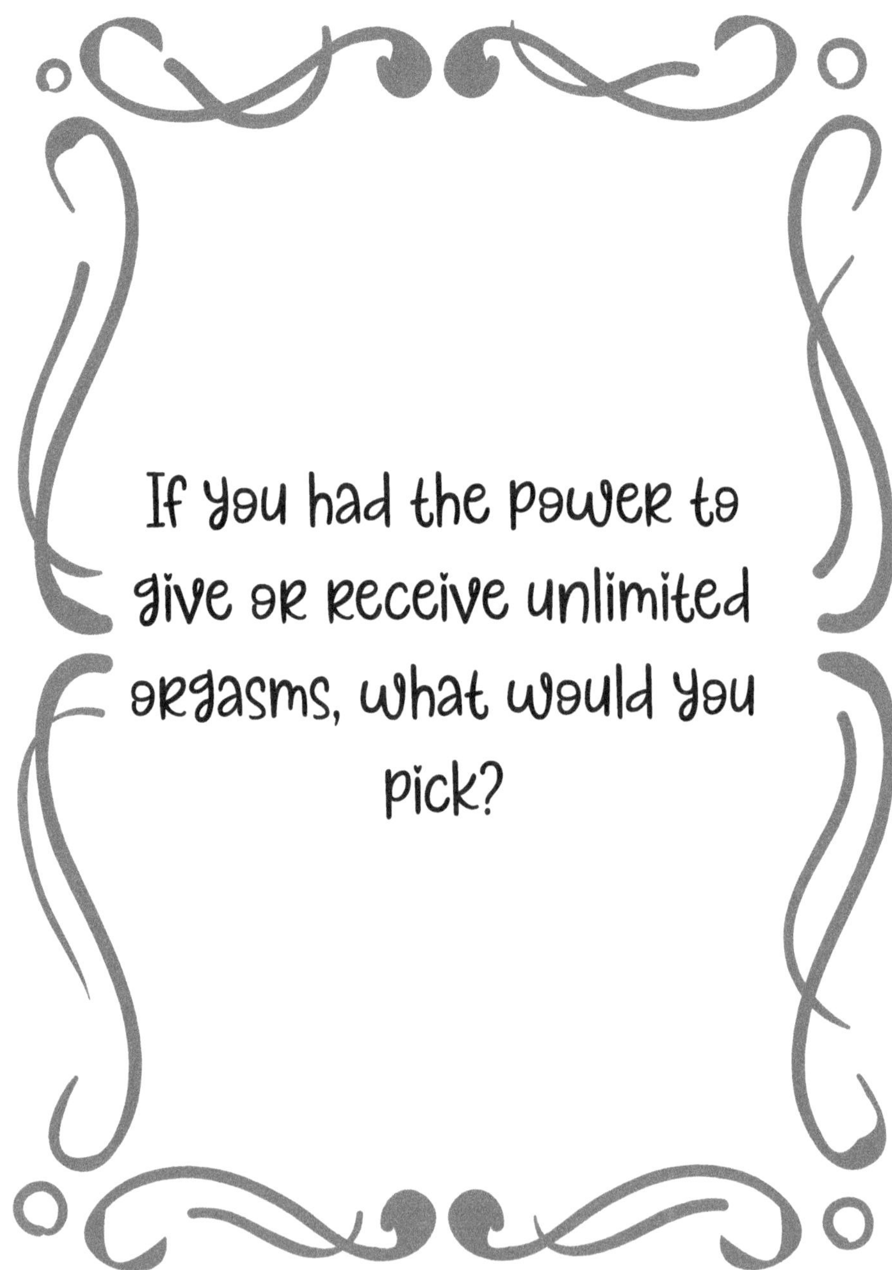

If you had the power to give or receive unlimited orgasms, what would you pick?

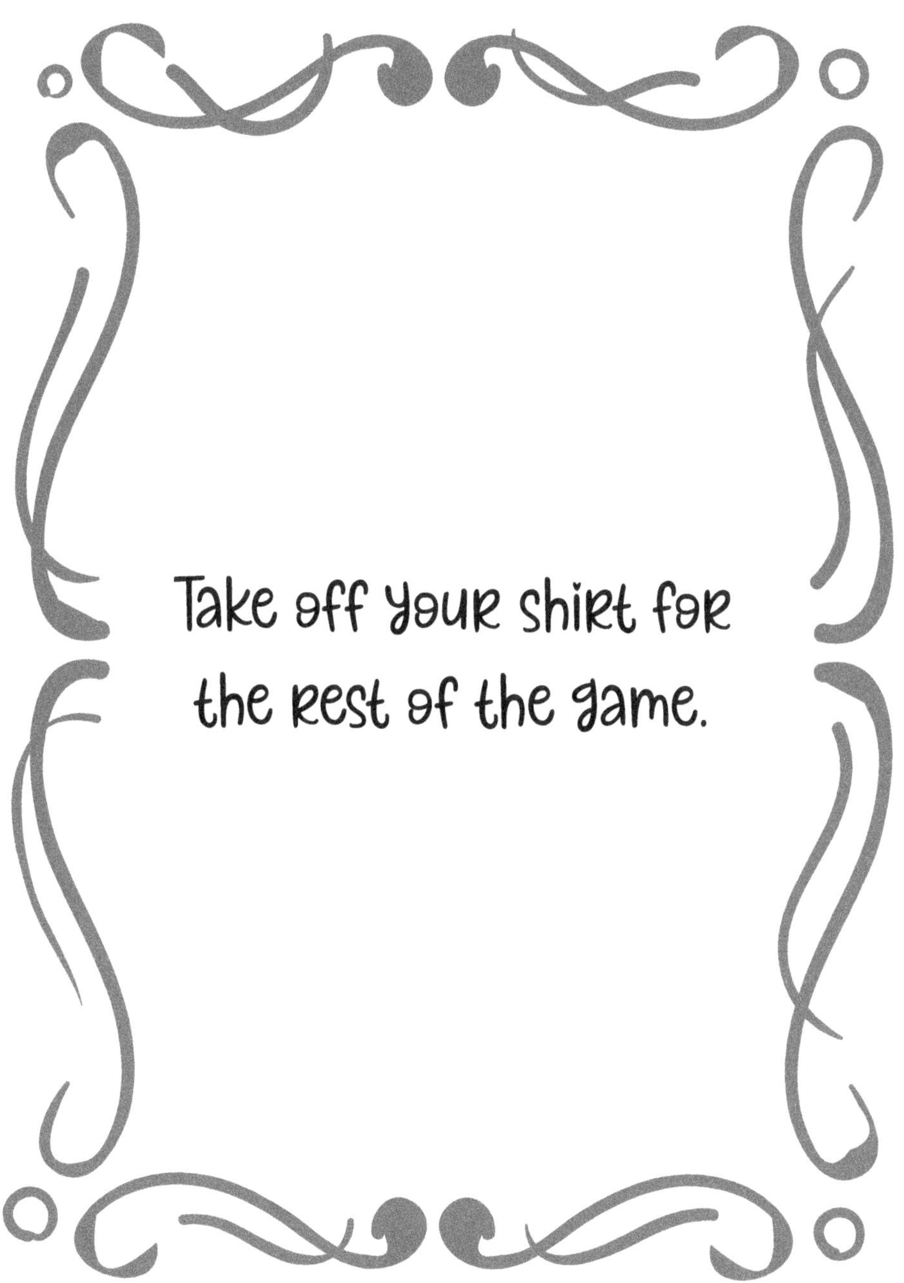

17
DARE

Take off your shirt for
the rest of the game.

DARE

#18

TRUTH

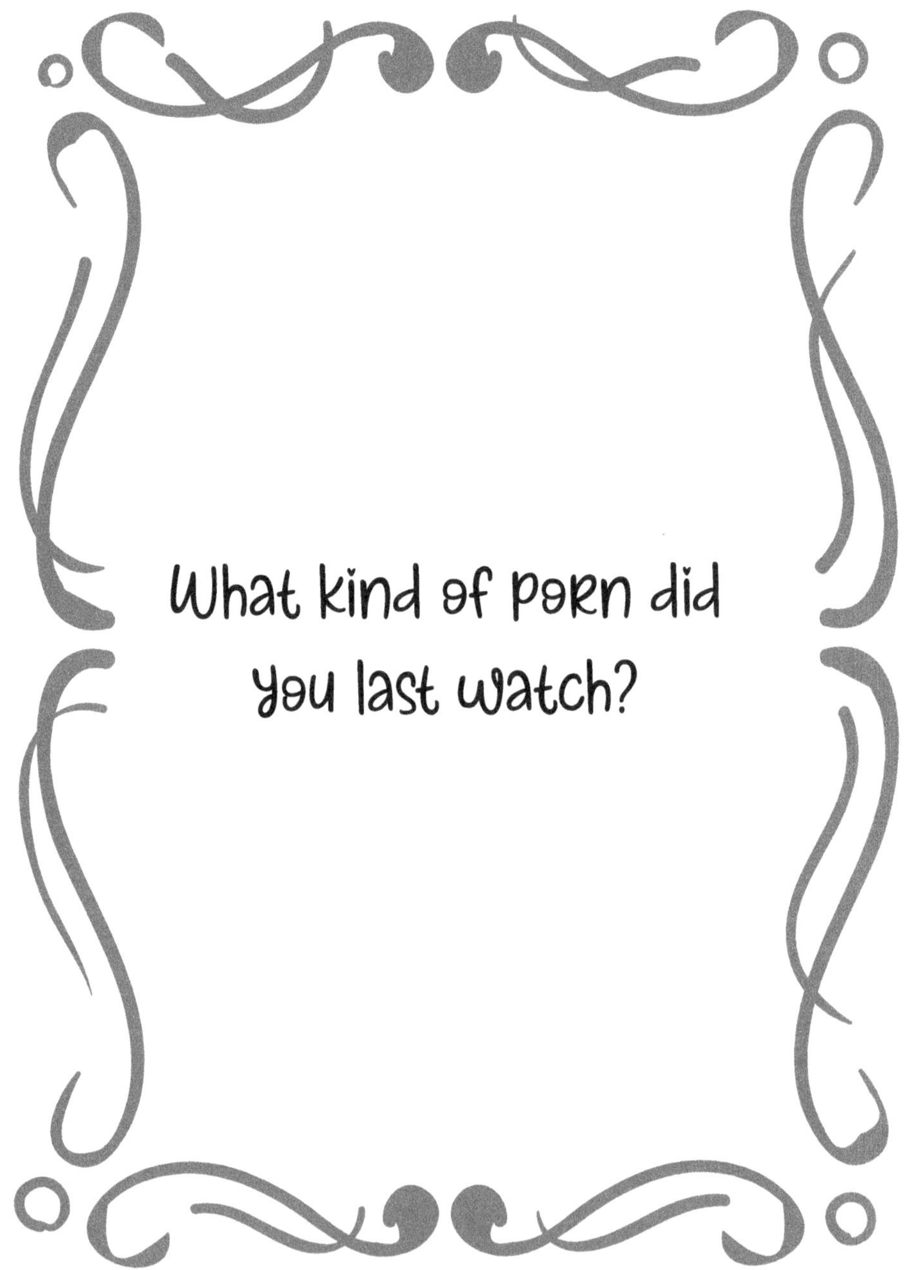

What kind of porn did
you last watch?

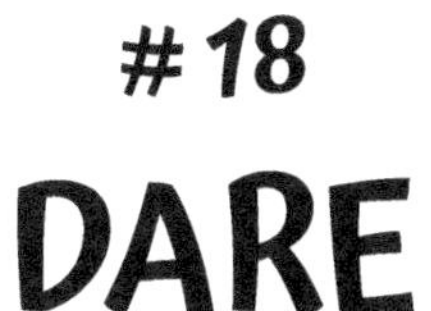

DARE

Take off your pants for
the rest of the game.

DARE

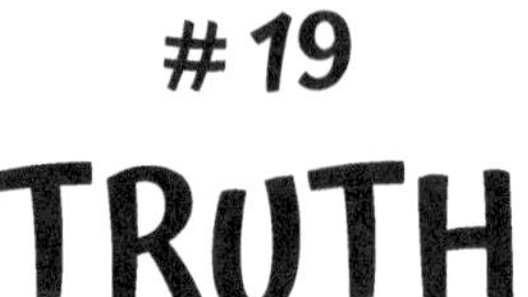

If you had to fuck one animal, what animal would you pick?

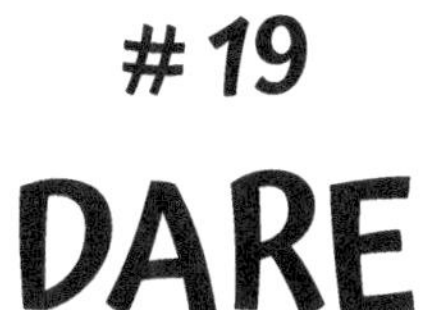

#19
DARE

Show me the sexiest picture you have on your phone.

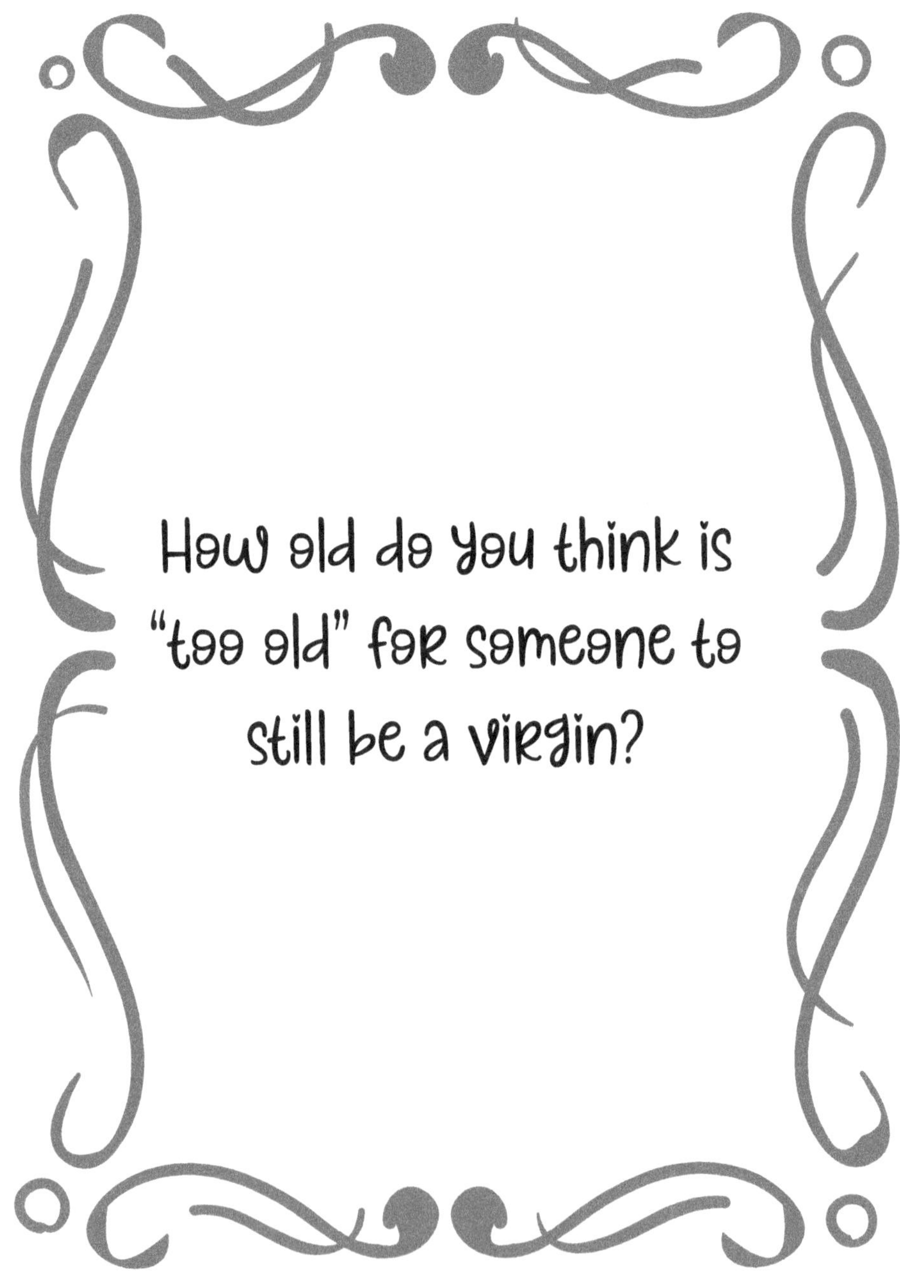

#20
TRUTH

How old do you think is "too old" for someone to still be a virgin?

20
DARE

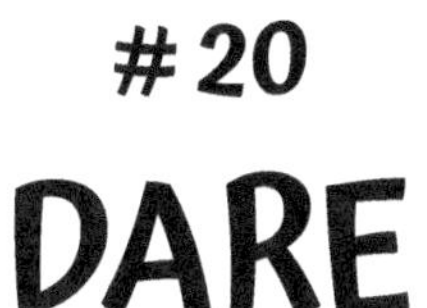

Put whipped cream on a
body part you want me to
lick it off of.

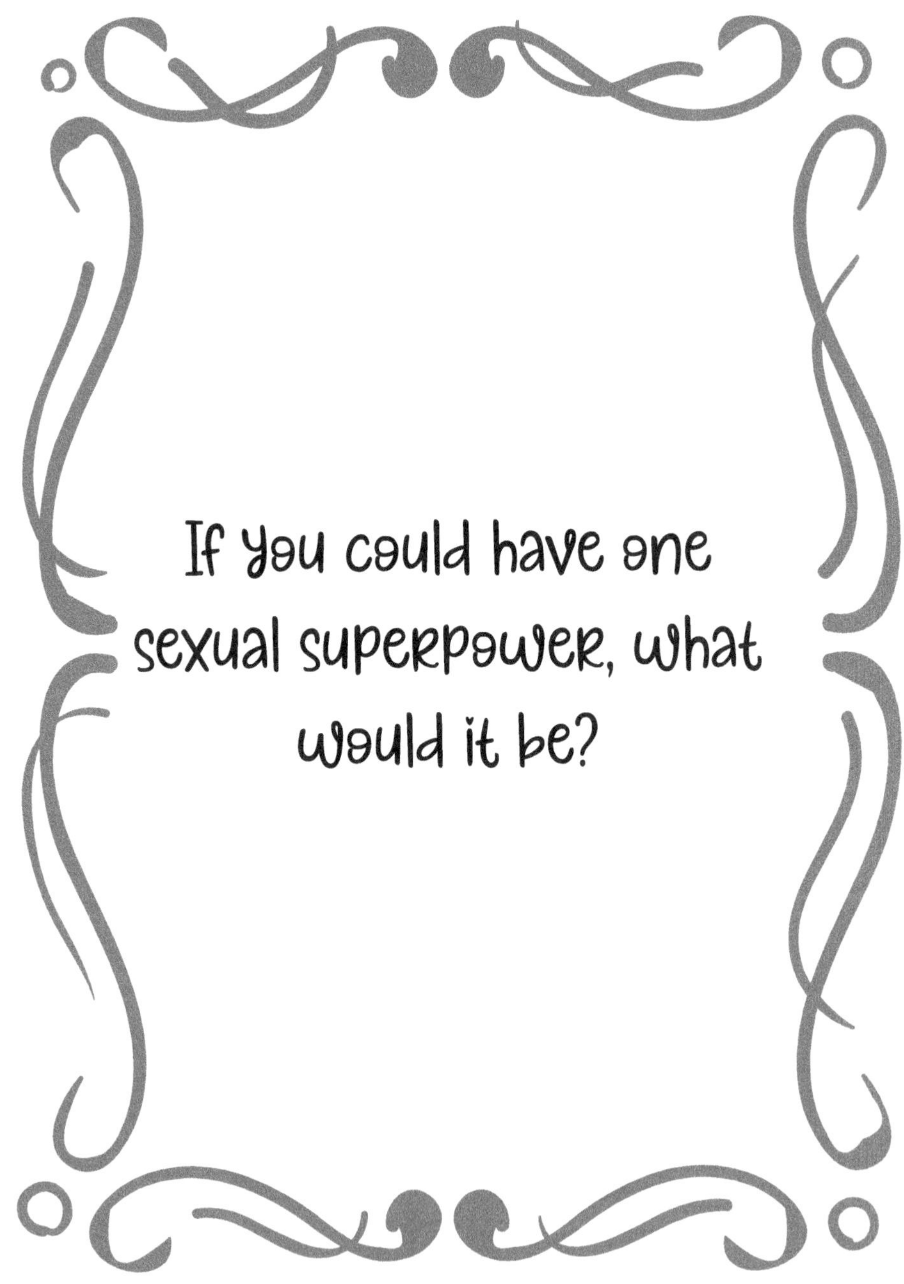

21
TRUTH

If you could have one sexual superpower, what would it be?

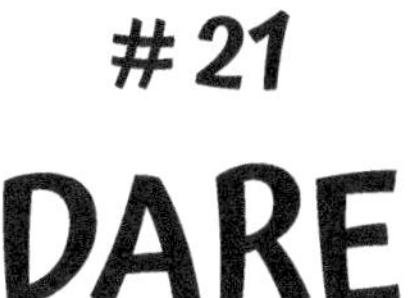

DARE

Fuck me in a room where we've never had sex before.

DARE

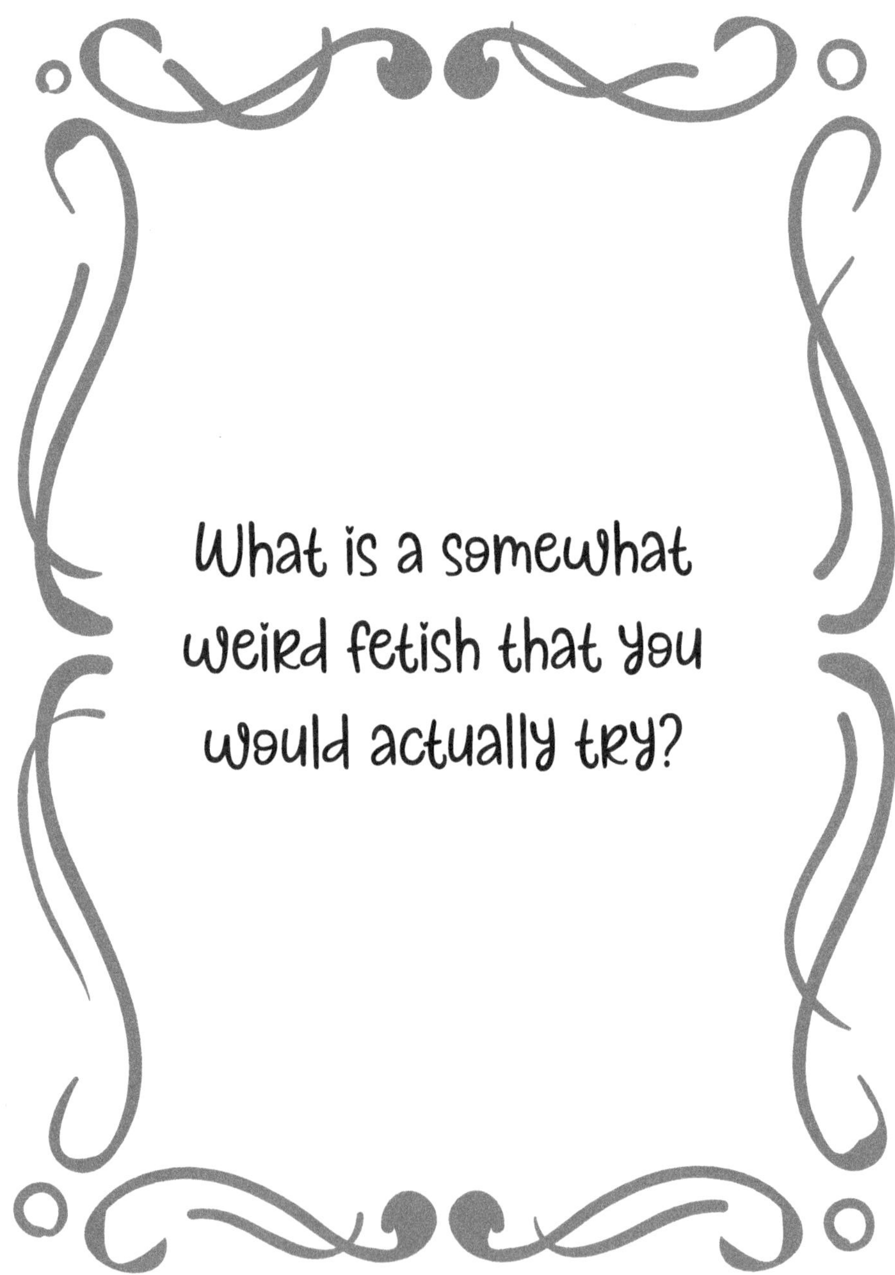

22
TRUTH

What is a somewhat weird fetish that you would actually try?

22
DARE

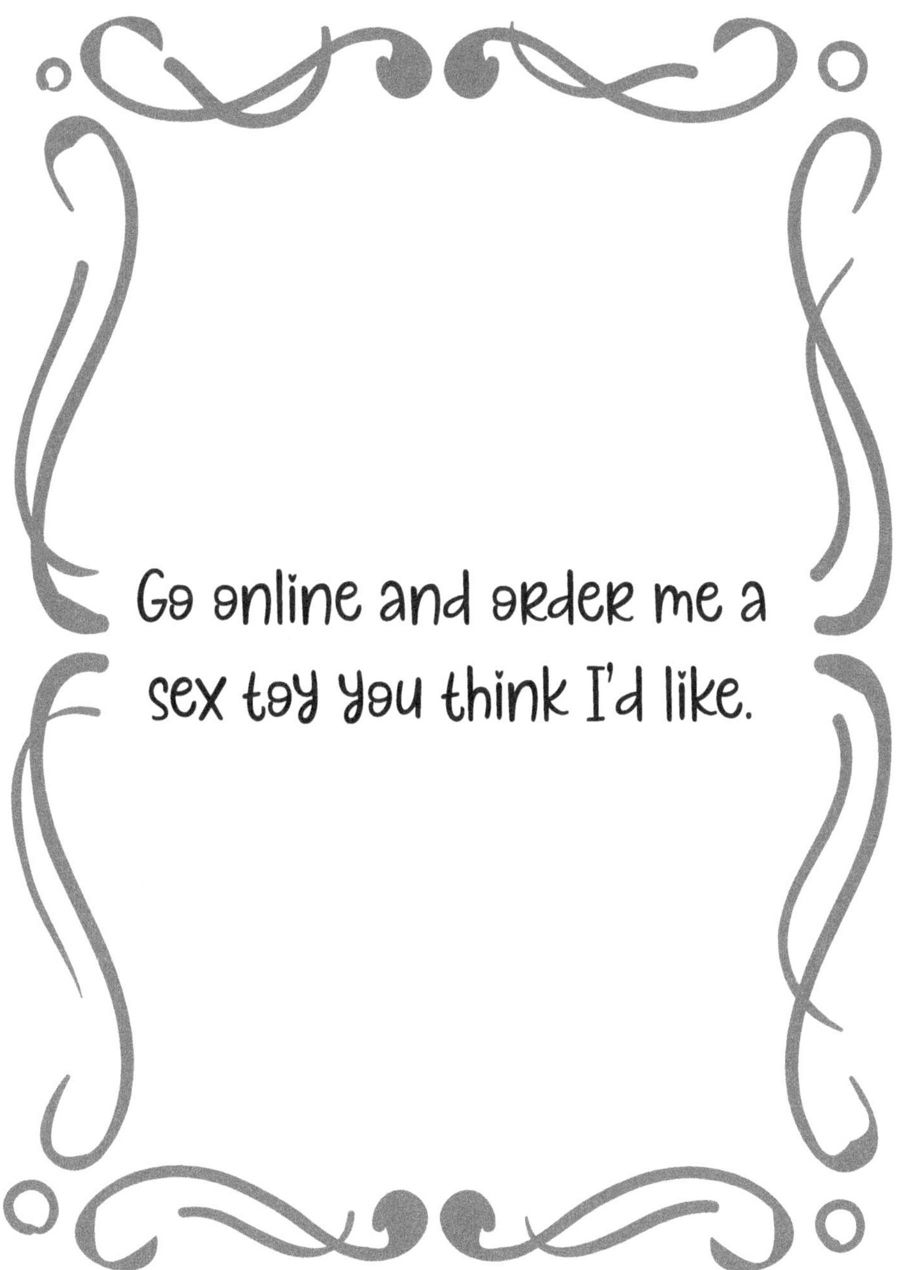

Go online and order me a
sex toy you think I'd like.

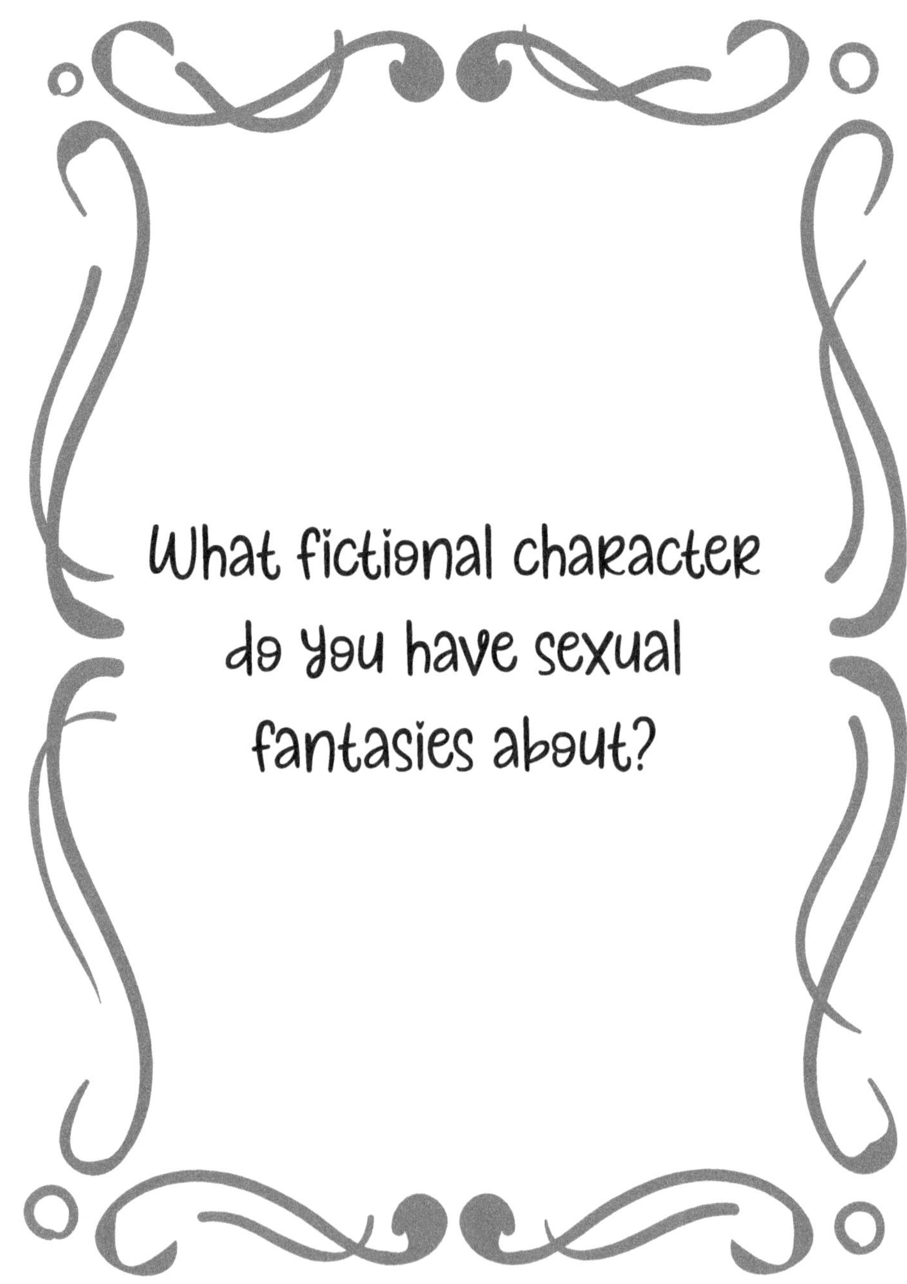

#23
TRUTH

What fictional character do you have sexual fantasies about?

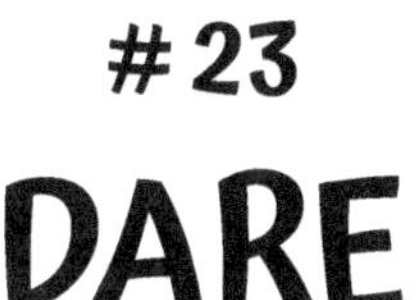

DARE

Show me a porn video you'd want us to act out together.

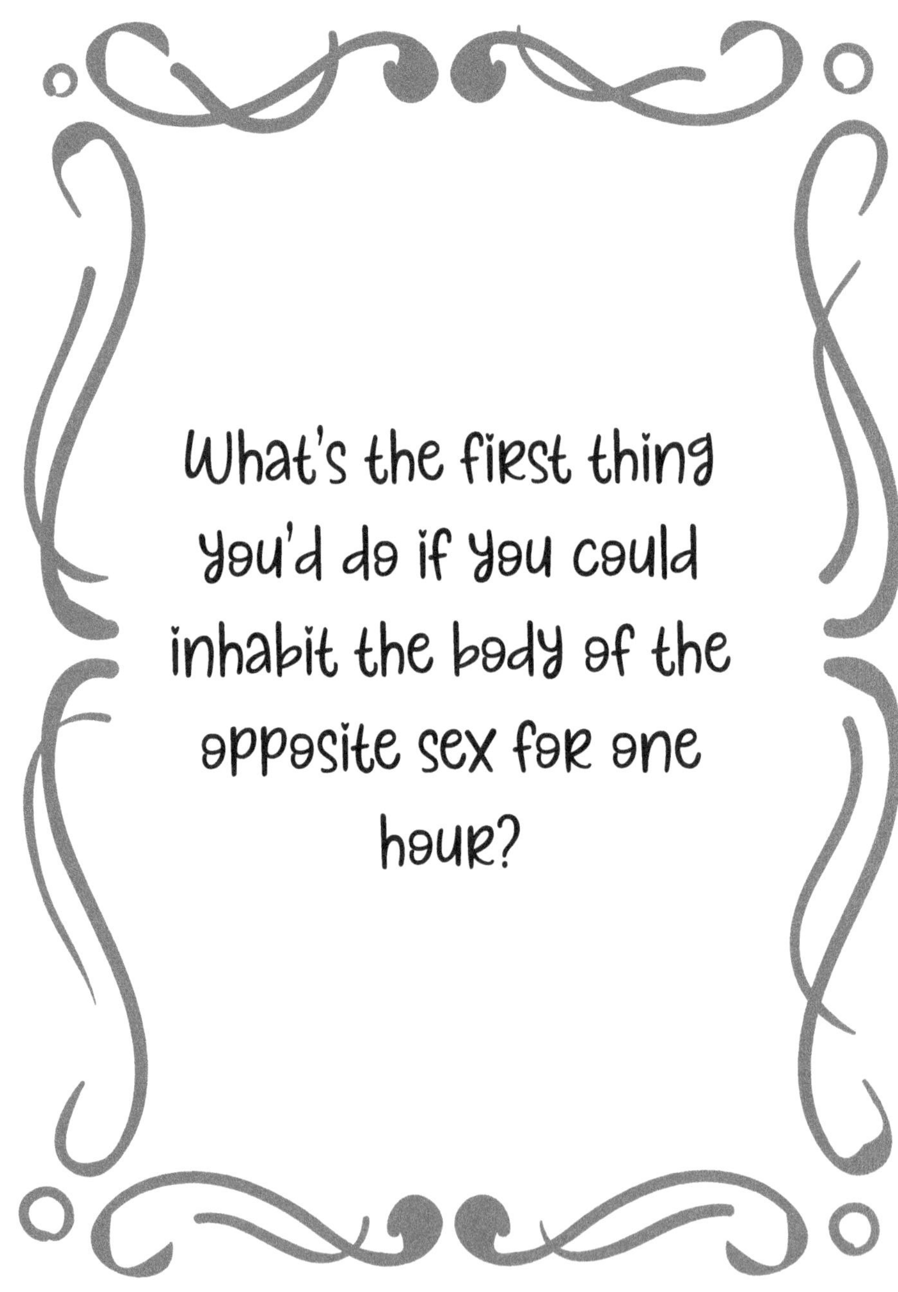

24
TRUTH

What's the first thing you'd do if you could inhabit the body of the opposite sex for one hour?

#24
DARE

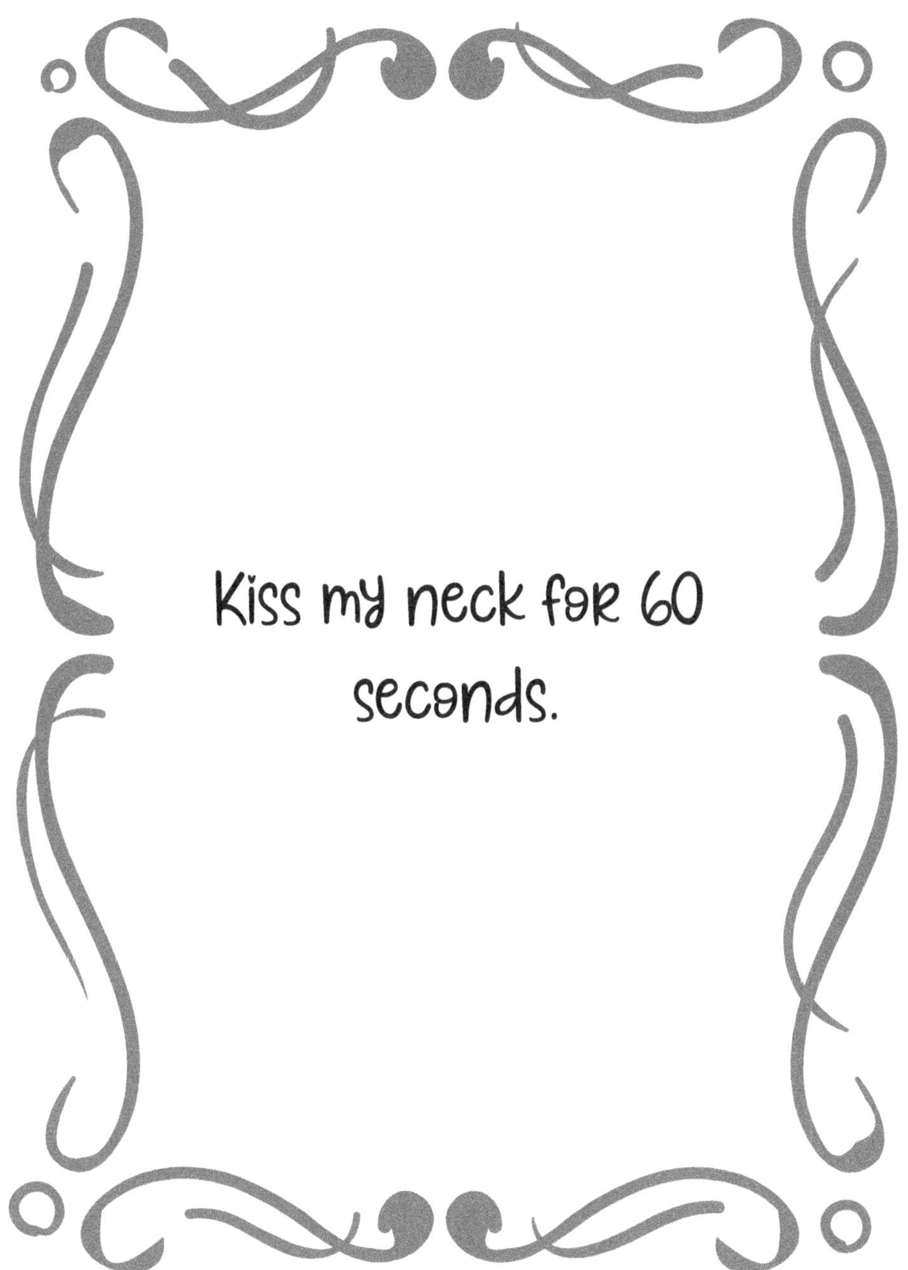

Kiss my neck for 60
seconds.

#25
TRUTH

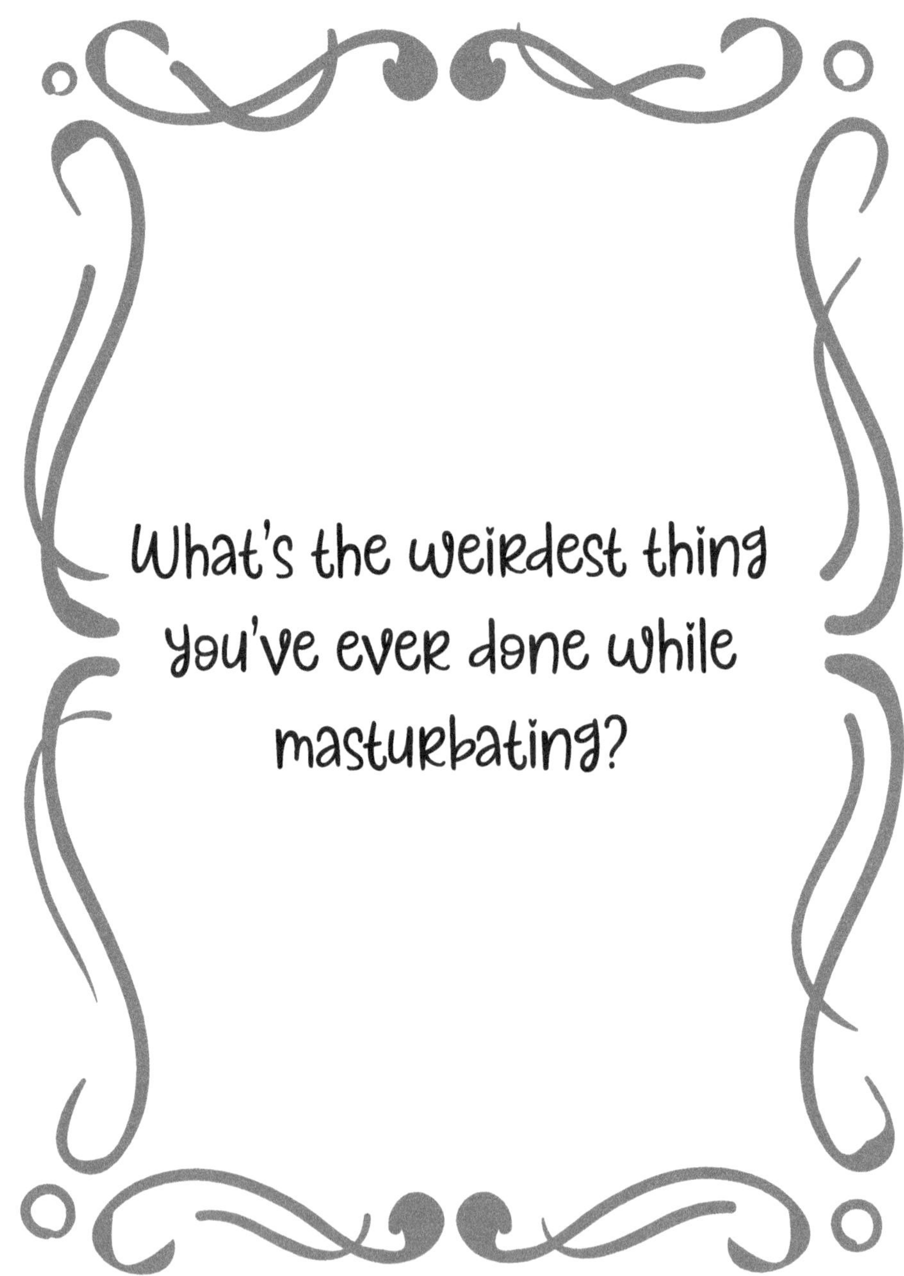

What's the weirdest thing you've ever done while masturbating?

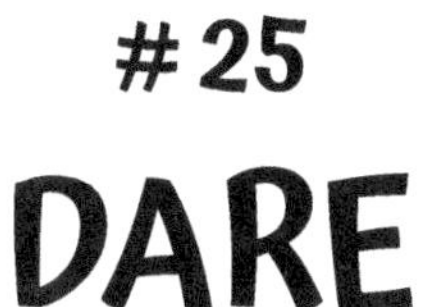

Do your best to try to make me orgasm in the next 5 minutes.

TRUTH

If you had to choose between having sex with one person for the rest of your life or never being able to have sex with the same person more than once, what would you pick?

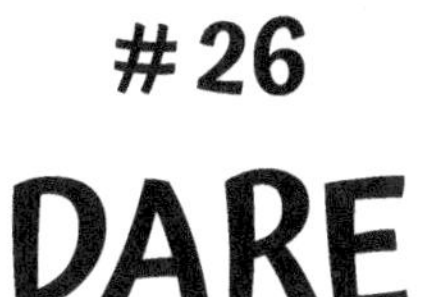

#26
DARE

Close your eyes and describe what my body looks like in detail.

TRUTH

Would you rather pay someone to put on a striptease for you (they aren't allowed to touch), pay someone to cuddle and massage you while wearing non-sexy clothes, or pay someone to talk dirty over the phone but never be able to see them?

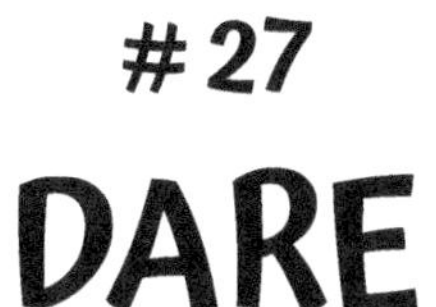

27
DARE

Try to get me aroused just by touching me, but without touching any sexual parts.

TRUTH

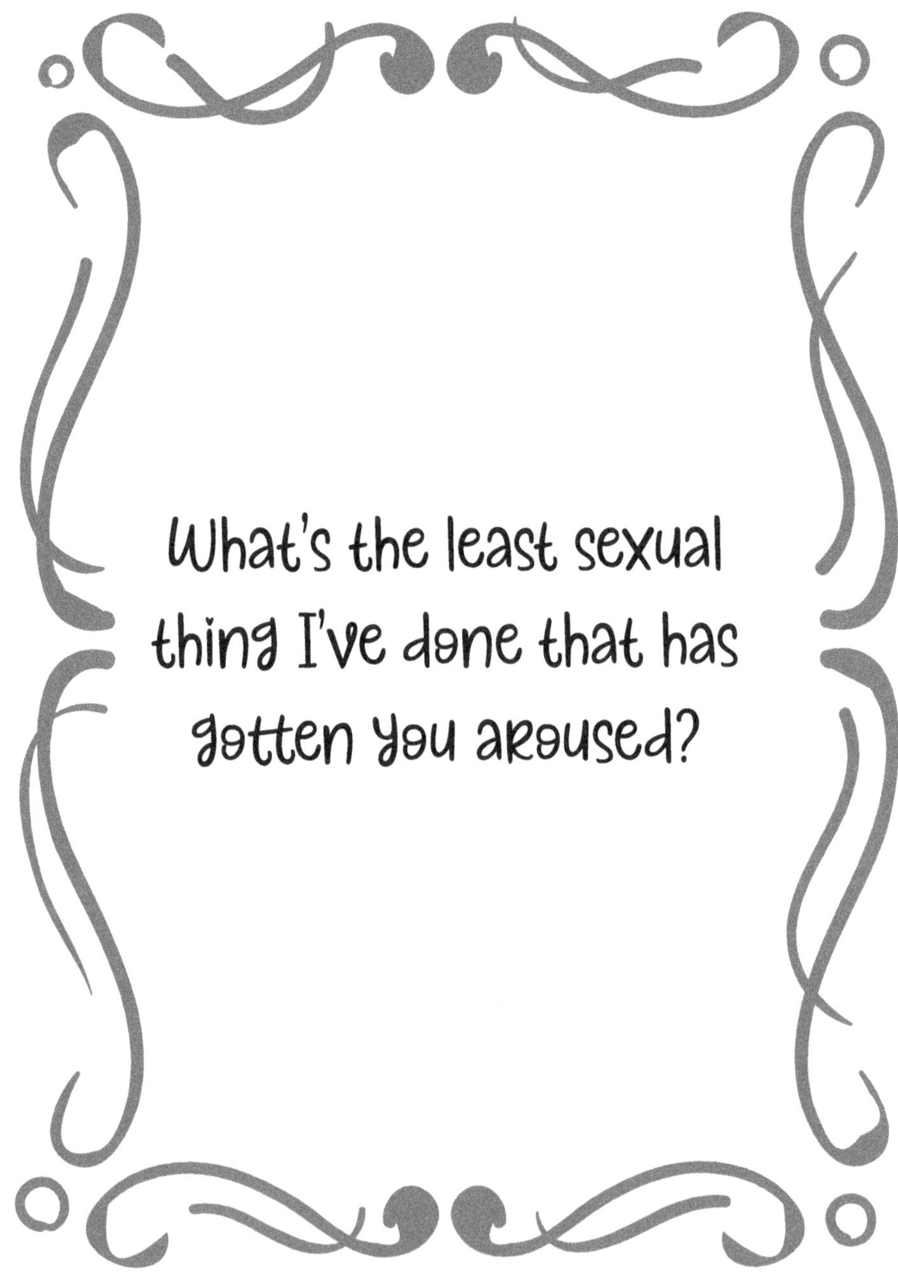

What's the least sexual thing I've done that has gotten you aroused?

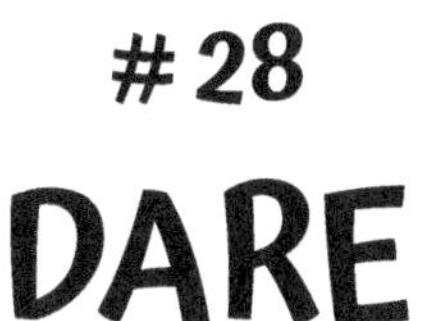

28
DARE

Whisper in my ear something you've always wanted to see me do in bed.

DARE

#29
TRUTH

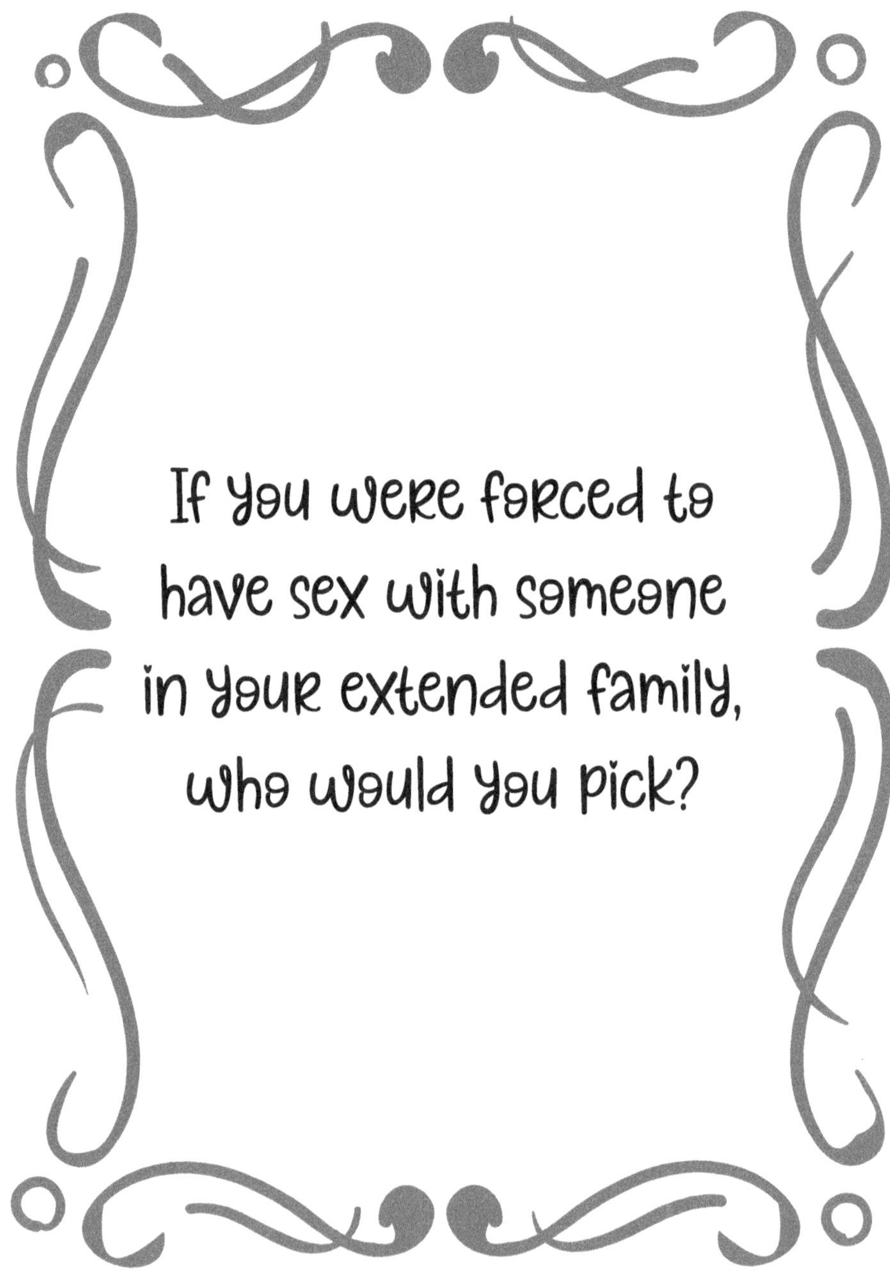

If you were forced to
have sex with someone
in your extended family,
who would you pick?

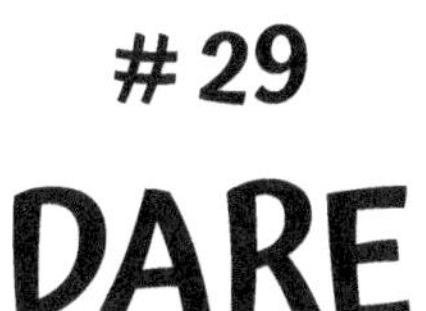

29
DARE

Use your tongue to spell
out a secret you have on
a part of my body.

30
TRUTH

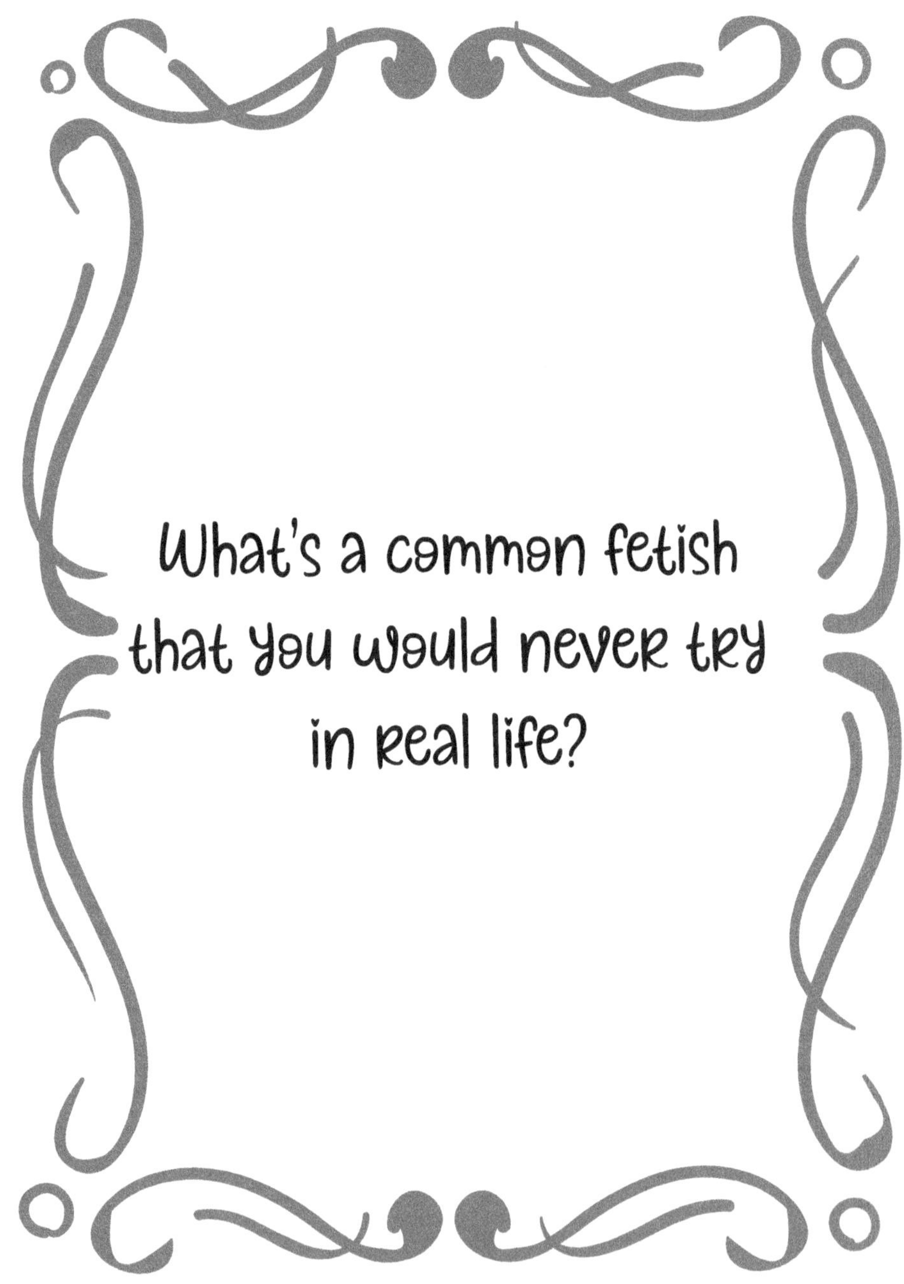

What's a common fetish that you would never try in real life?

#30
DARE

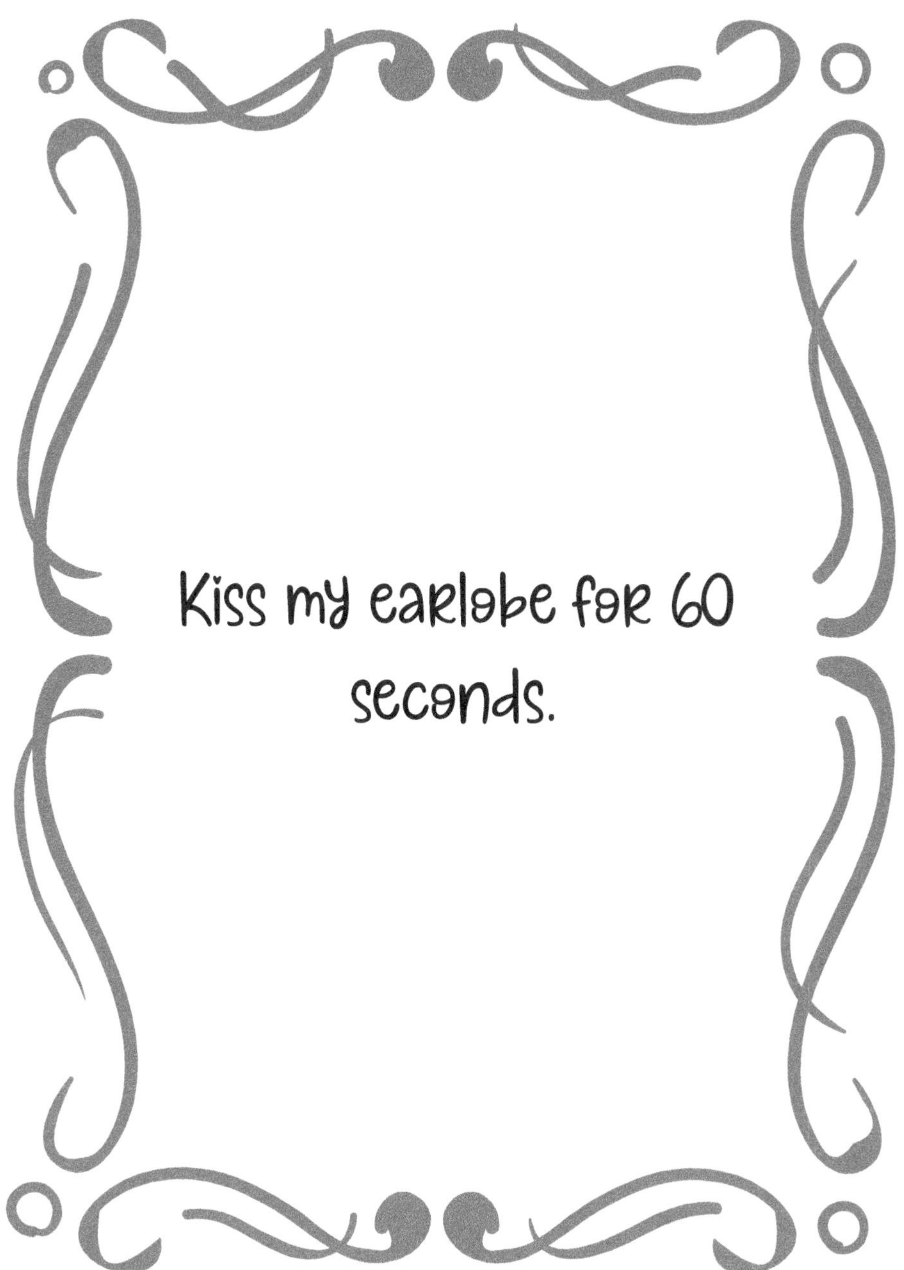

Kiss my earlobe for 60 seconds.

31
TRUTH

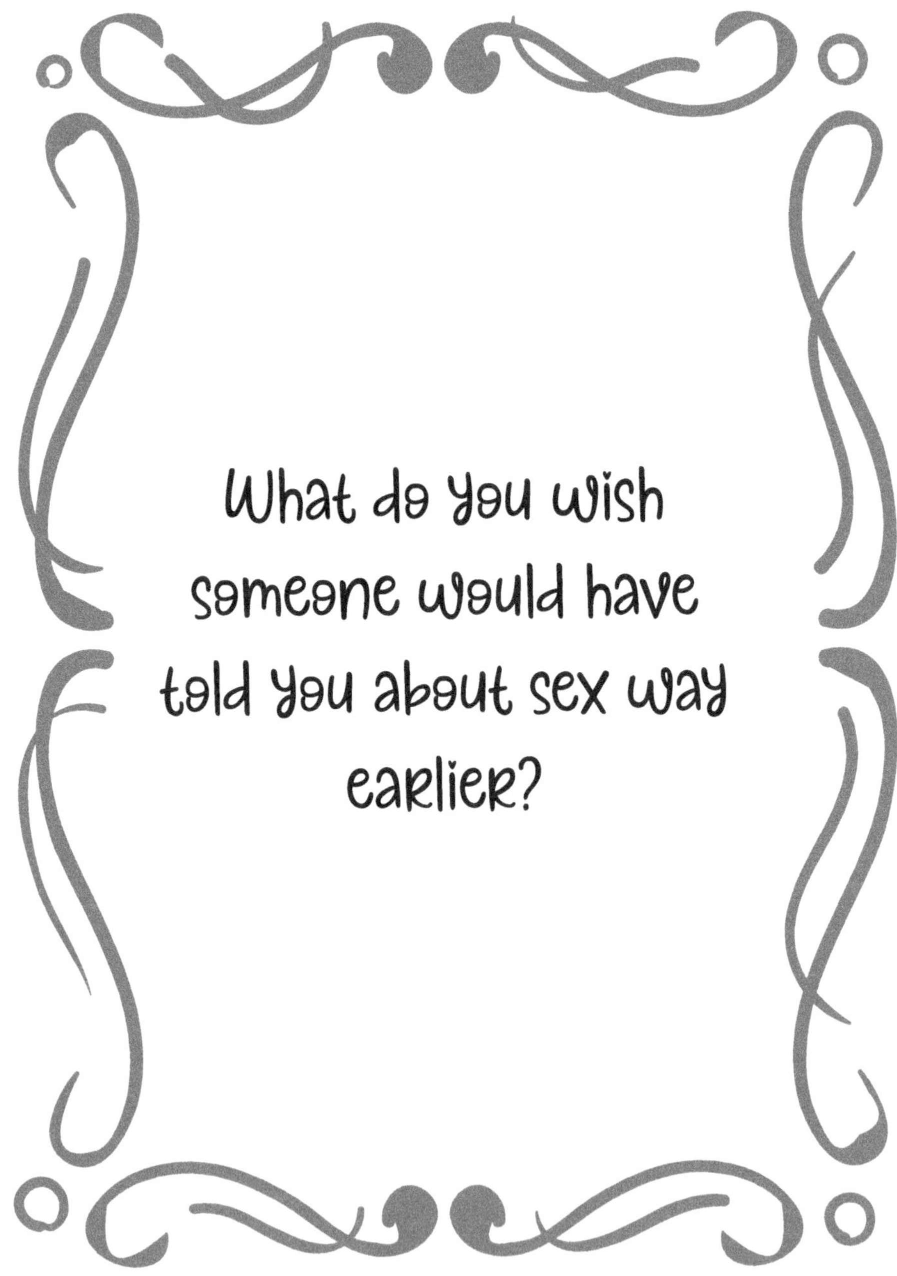

What do you wish
someone would have
told you about sex way
earlier?

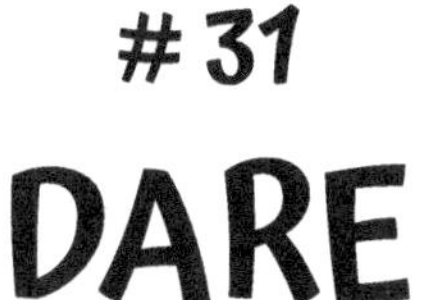

31
DARE

Put a blindfold on, stick your tongue out, and try to guess what I touch it with.

#32
TRUTH

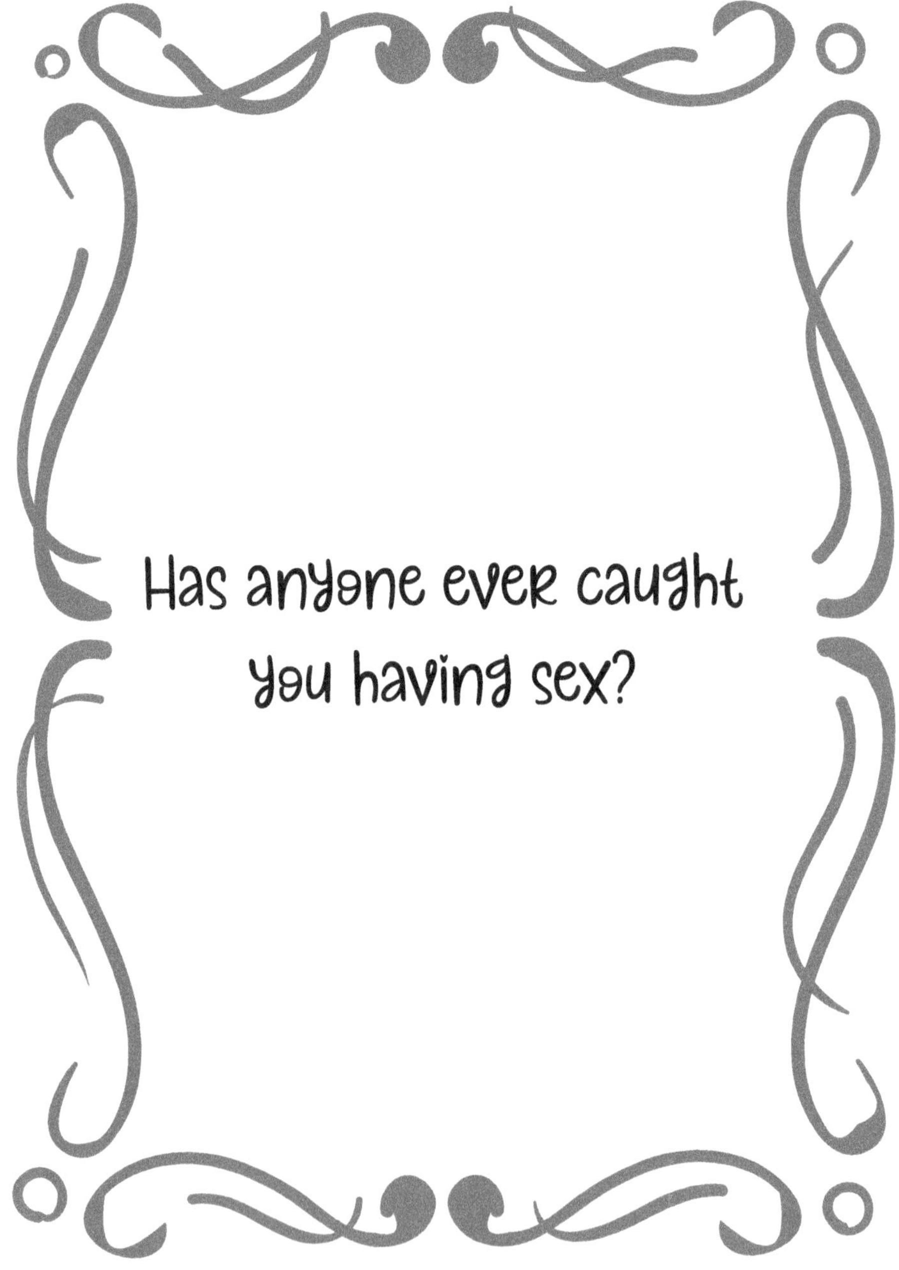

Has anyone ever caught
you having sex?

32
DARE

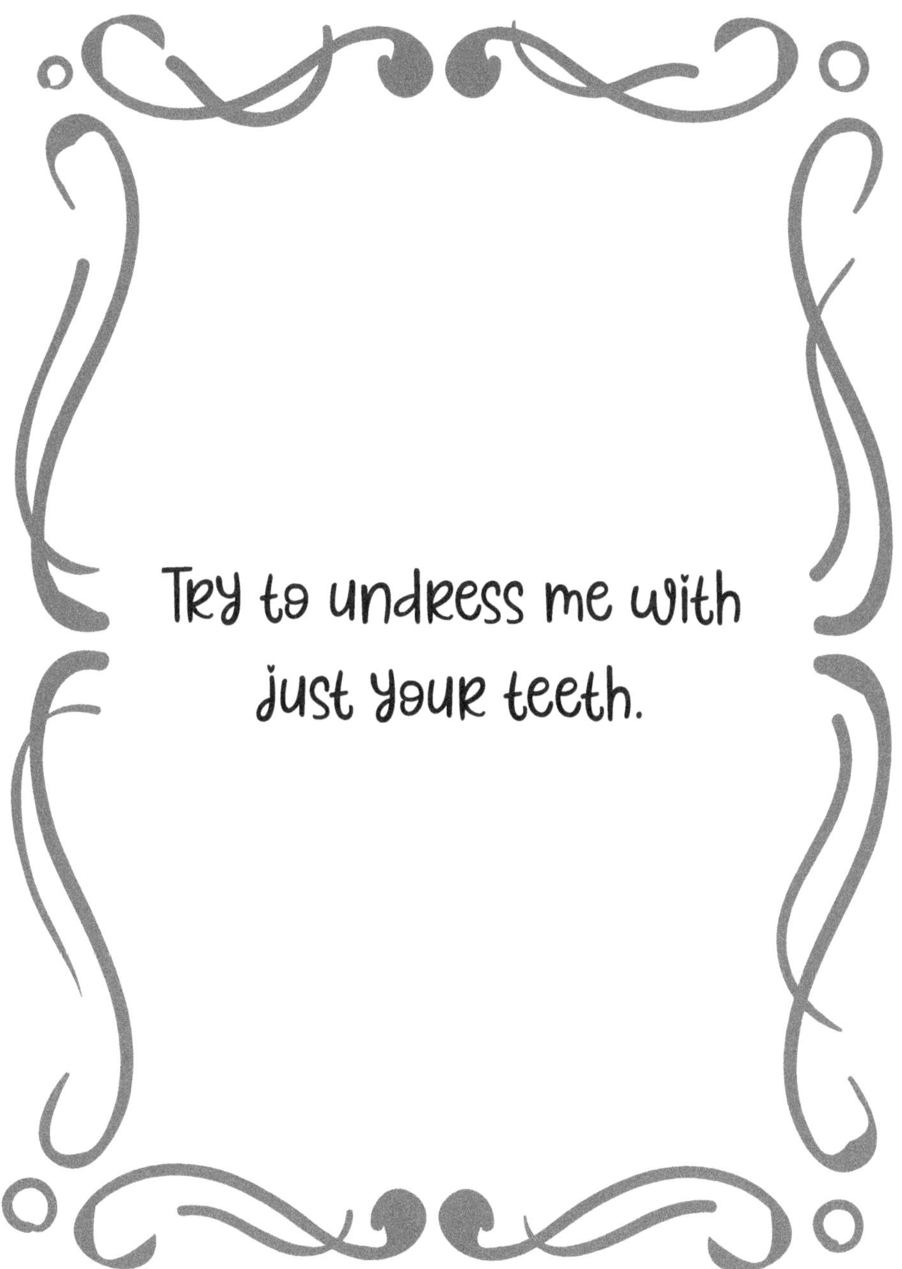

Try to undress me with
just your teeth.

33
TRUTH

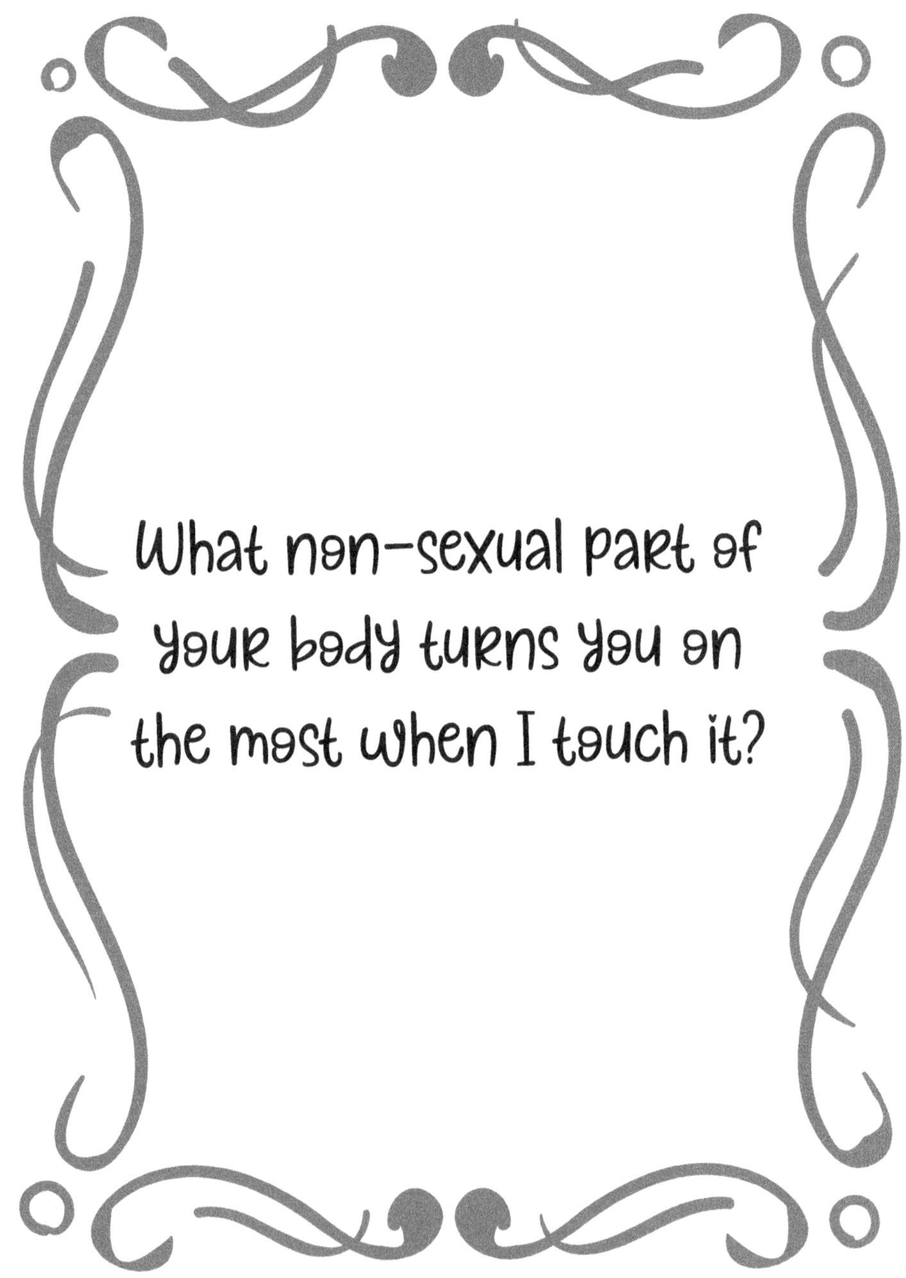

What non-sexual part of your body turns you on the most when I touch it?

#33
DARE

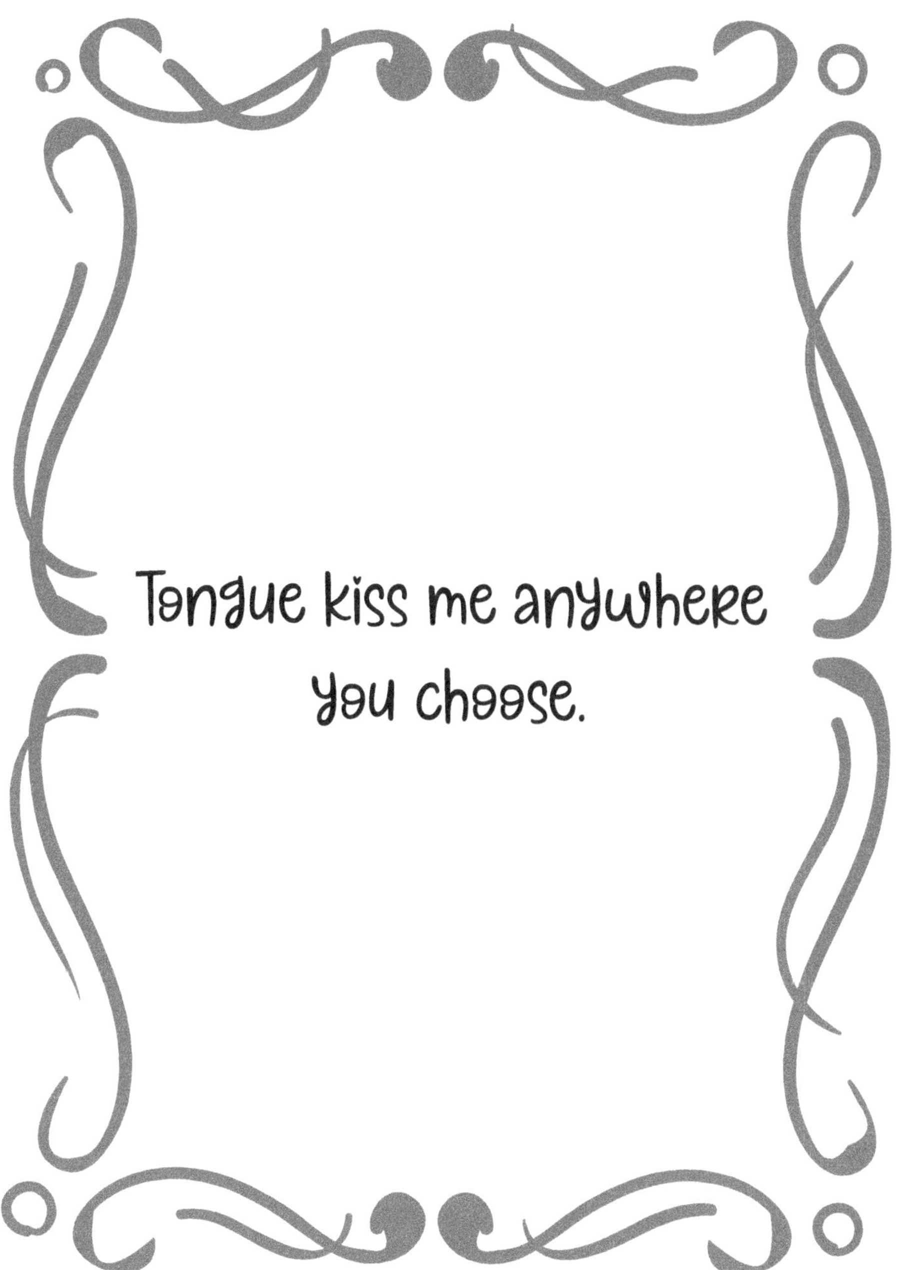

#34
TRUTH

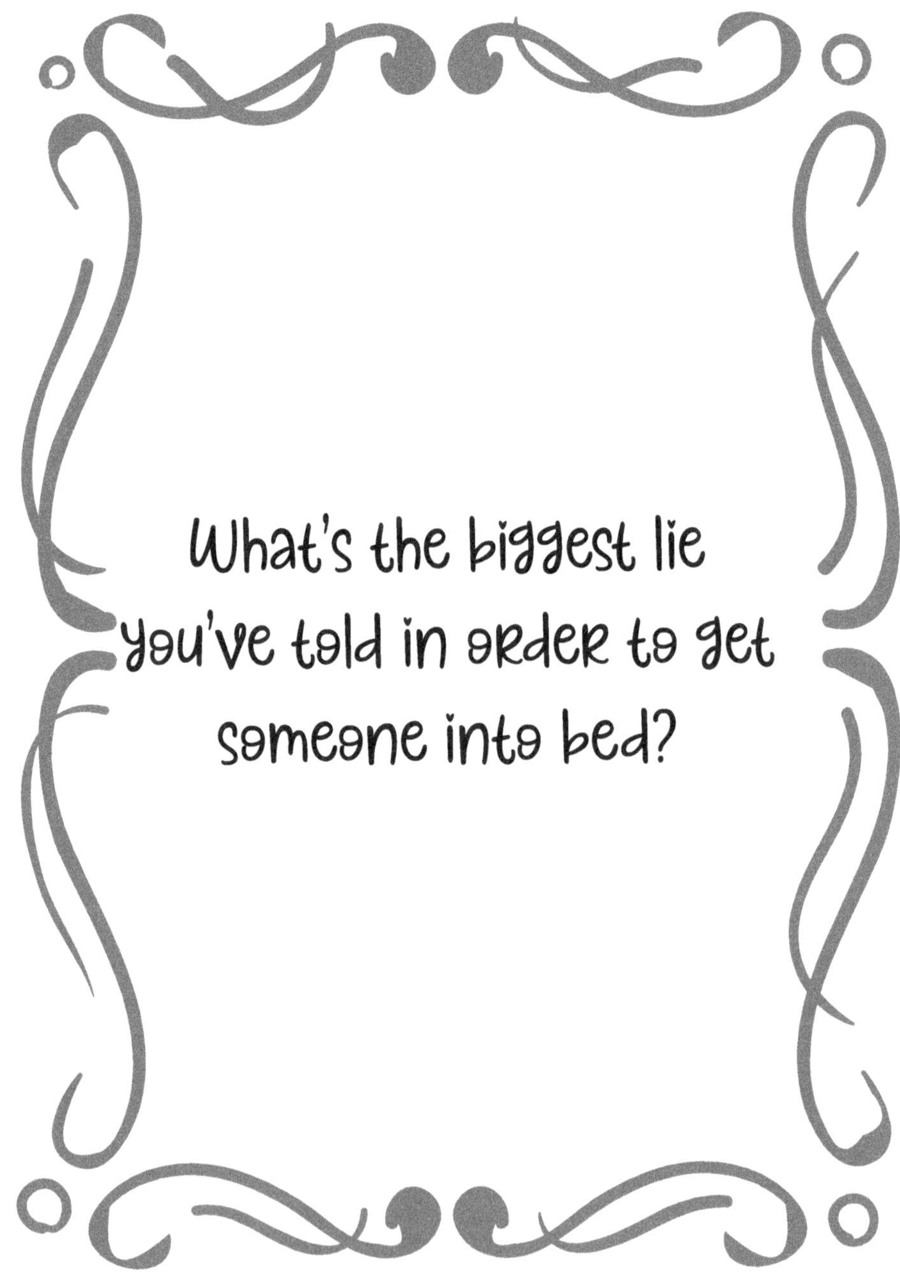

What's the biggest lie
you've told in order to get
someone into bed?

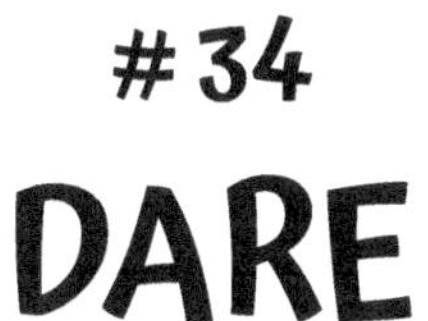

34

DARE

Try not to get turned
on while I sit on your lap
and kiss your neck for 60
seconds.

DARE

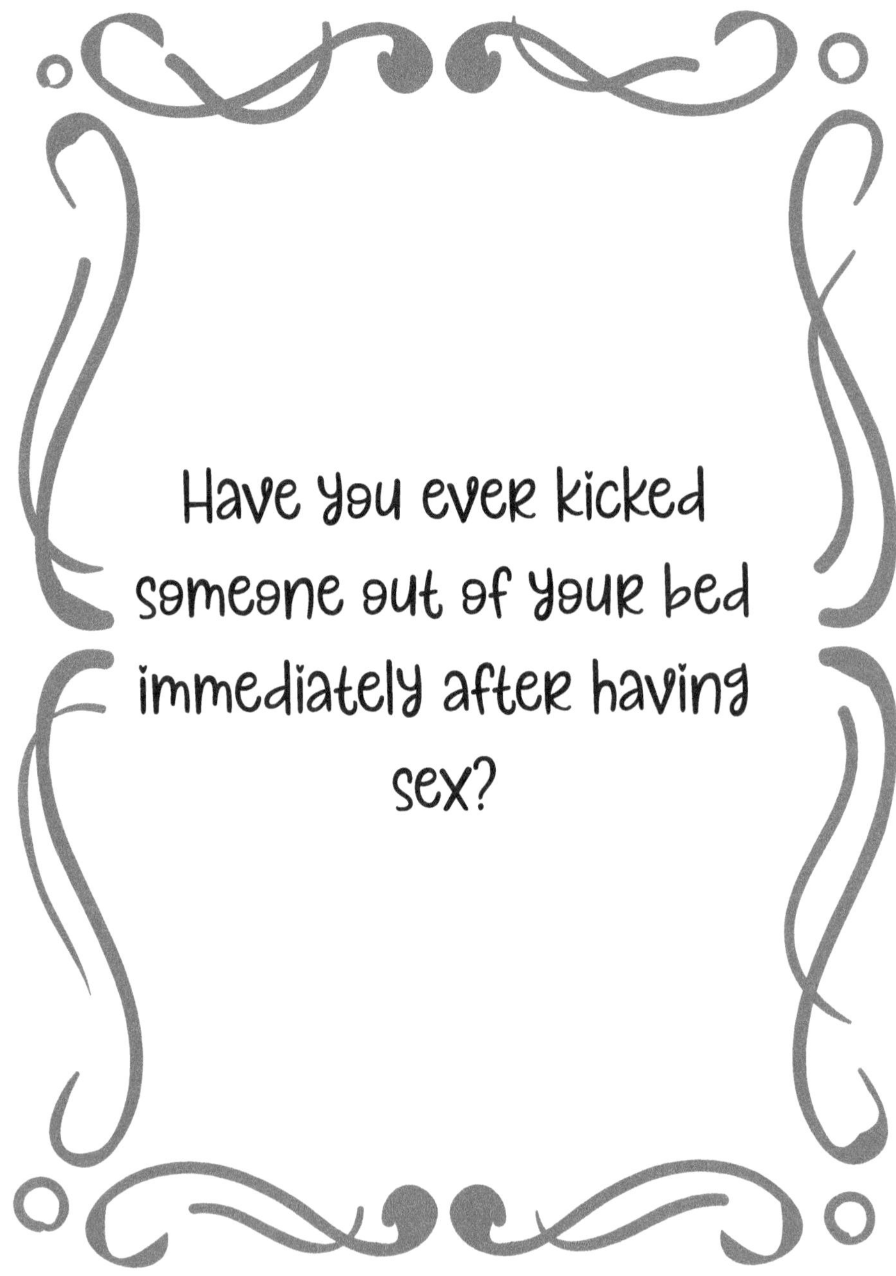

#35
TRUTH

Have you ever kicked someone out of your bed immediately after having sex?

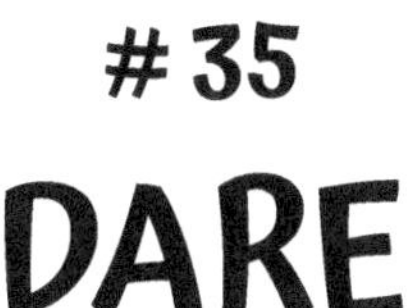

#35
DARE

Show me the dirtiest text message you have in your phone.

36

TRUTH

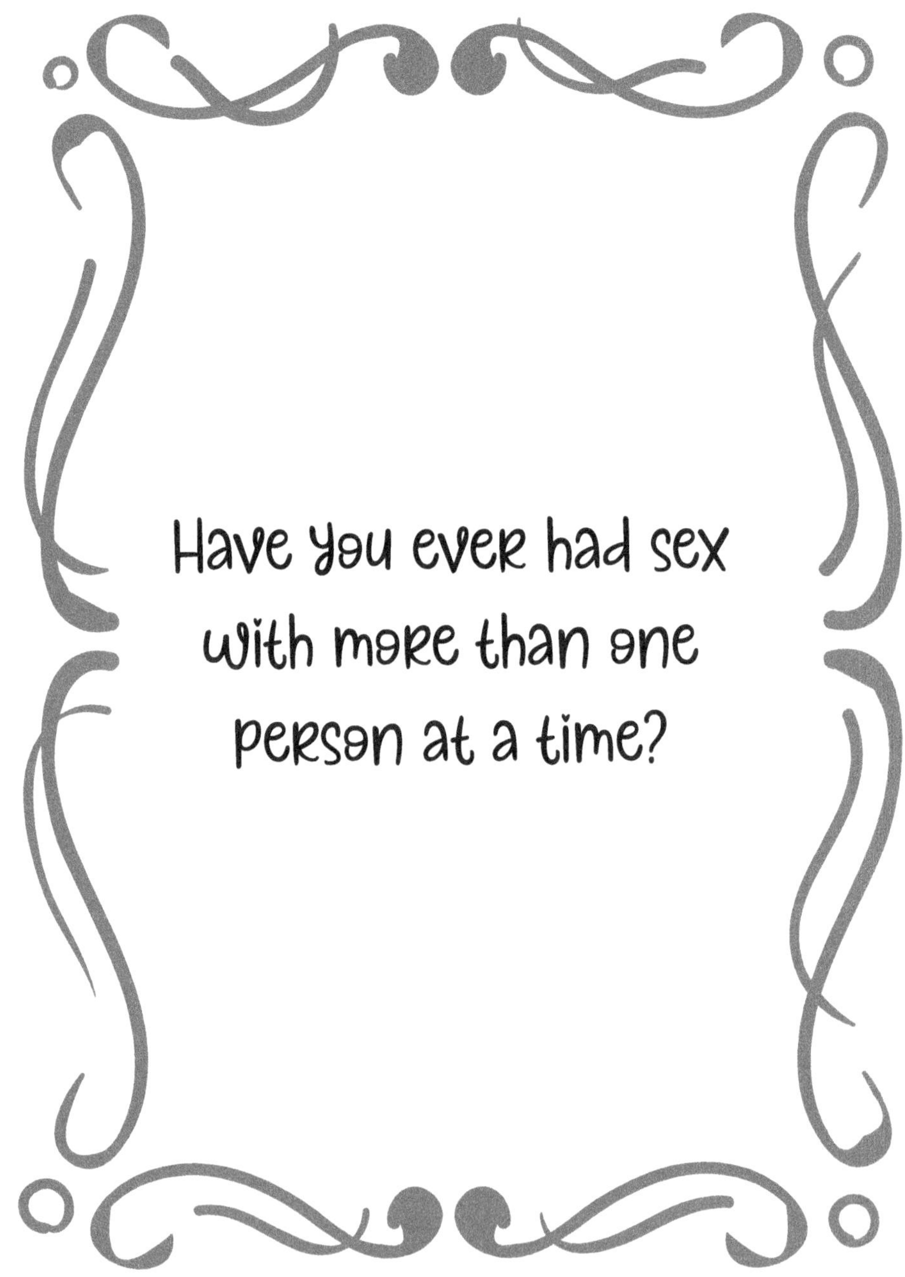

Have you ever had sex
with more than one
person at a time?

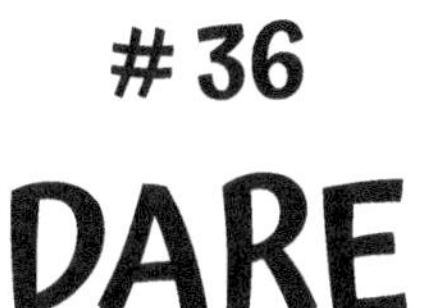

DARE

Whisper in my ear a sexy nickname you've never called me but always wanted to try.

37

TRUTH

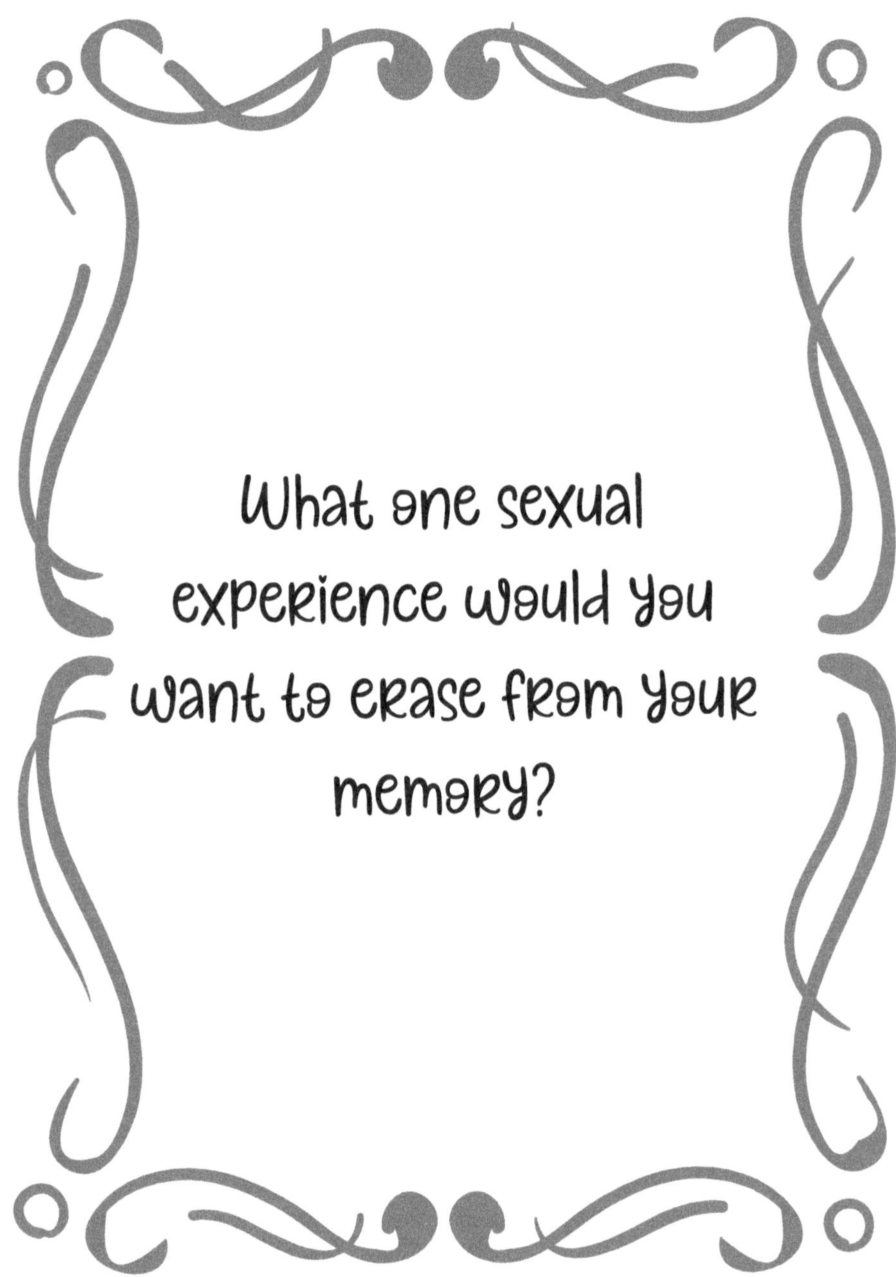

What one sexual
experience would you
want to erase from your
memory?

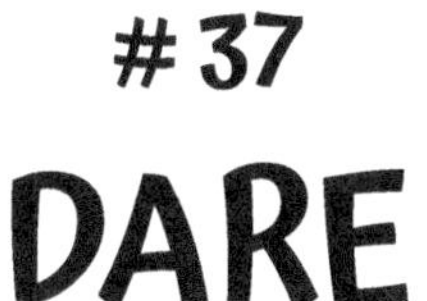

37
DARE

Go get something from the fridge and eat it as seductively as possible.

38

TRUTH

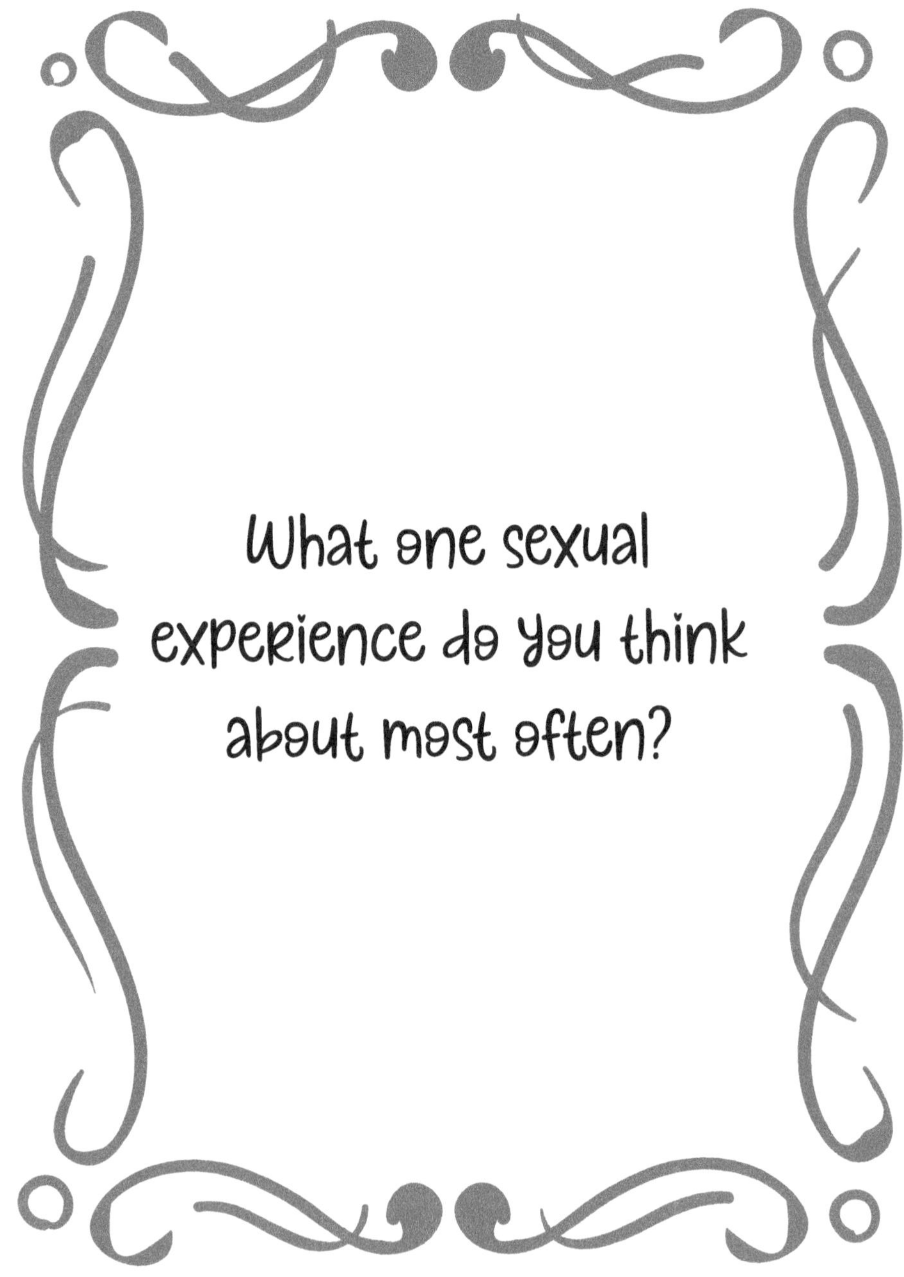

38
DARE

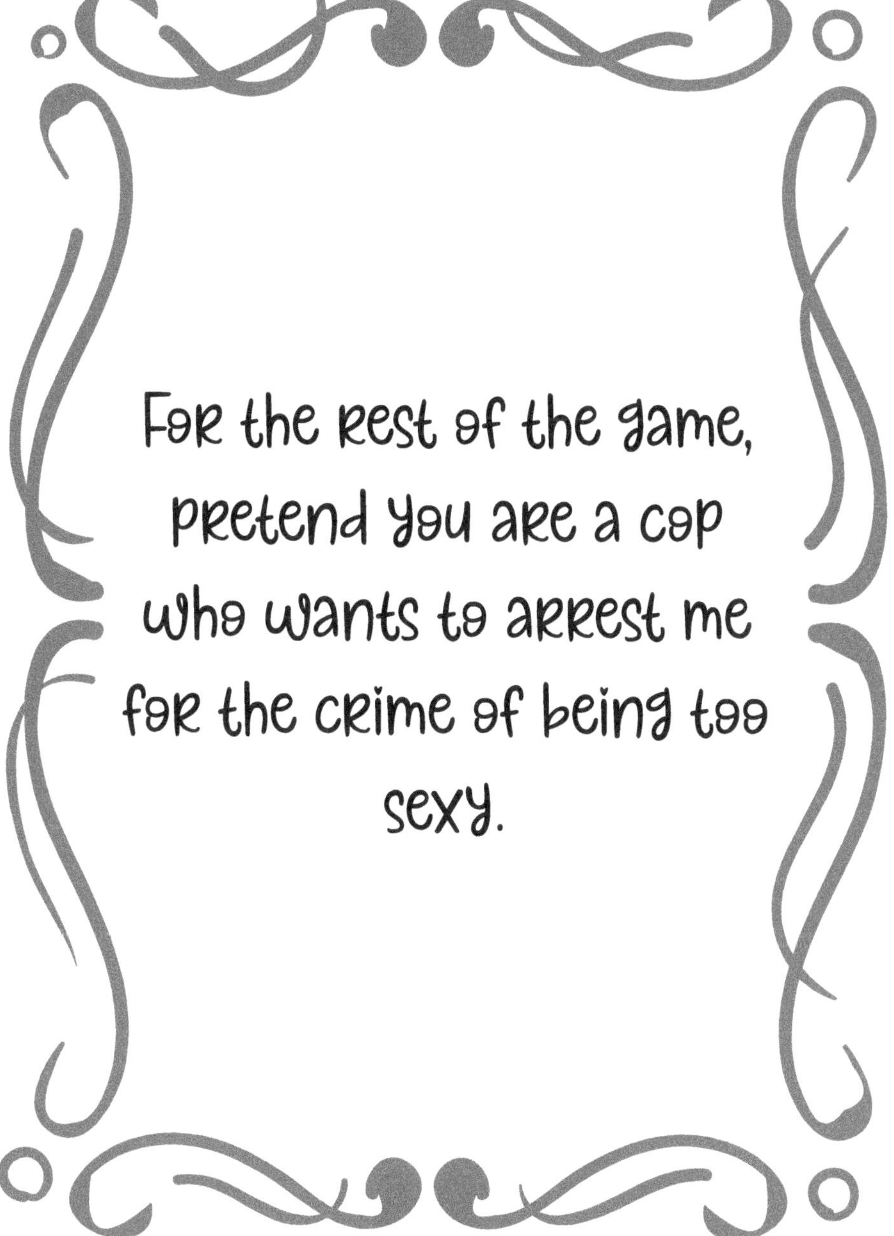

For the rest of the game, pretend you are a cop who wants to arrest me for the crime of being too sexy.

#39
TRUTH

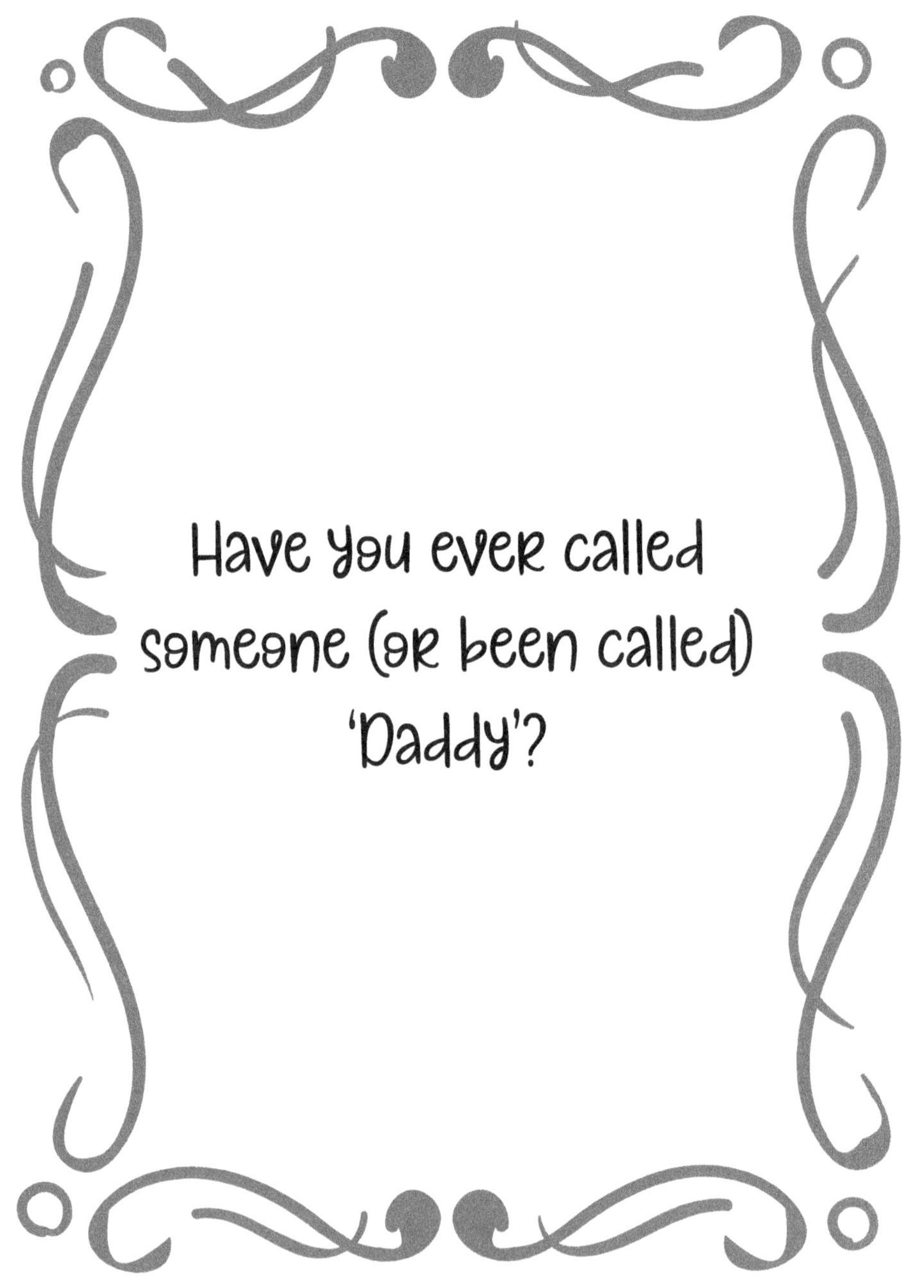

Have you ever called
someone (or been called)
'Daddy'?

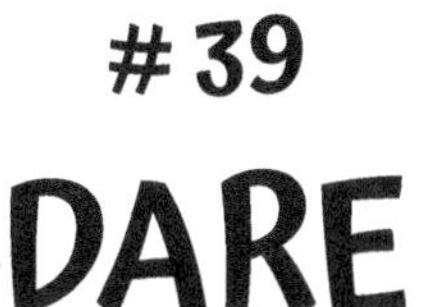

39
DARE

Show me with your hands what you want my tongue to do.

#40
TRUTH

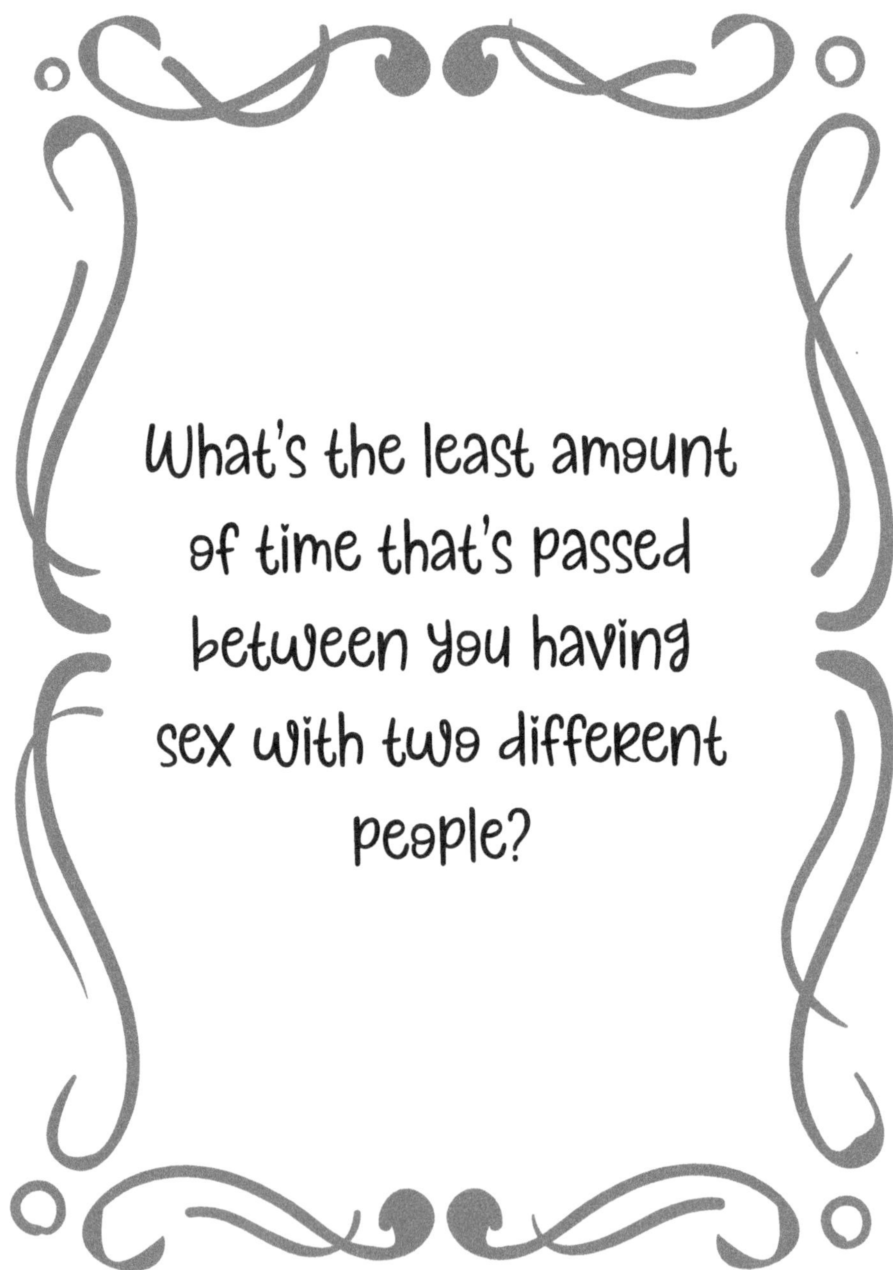

What's the least amount of time that's passed between you having sex with two different people?

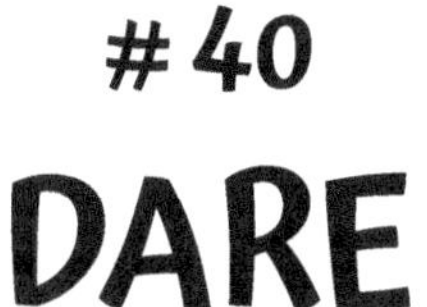

DARE

Try to turn me on using touch, but you can only touch my arms and hands.

DARE

#41
TRUTH

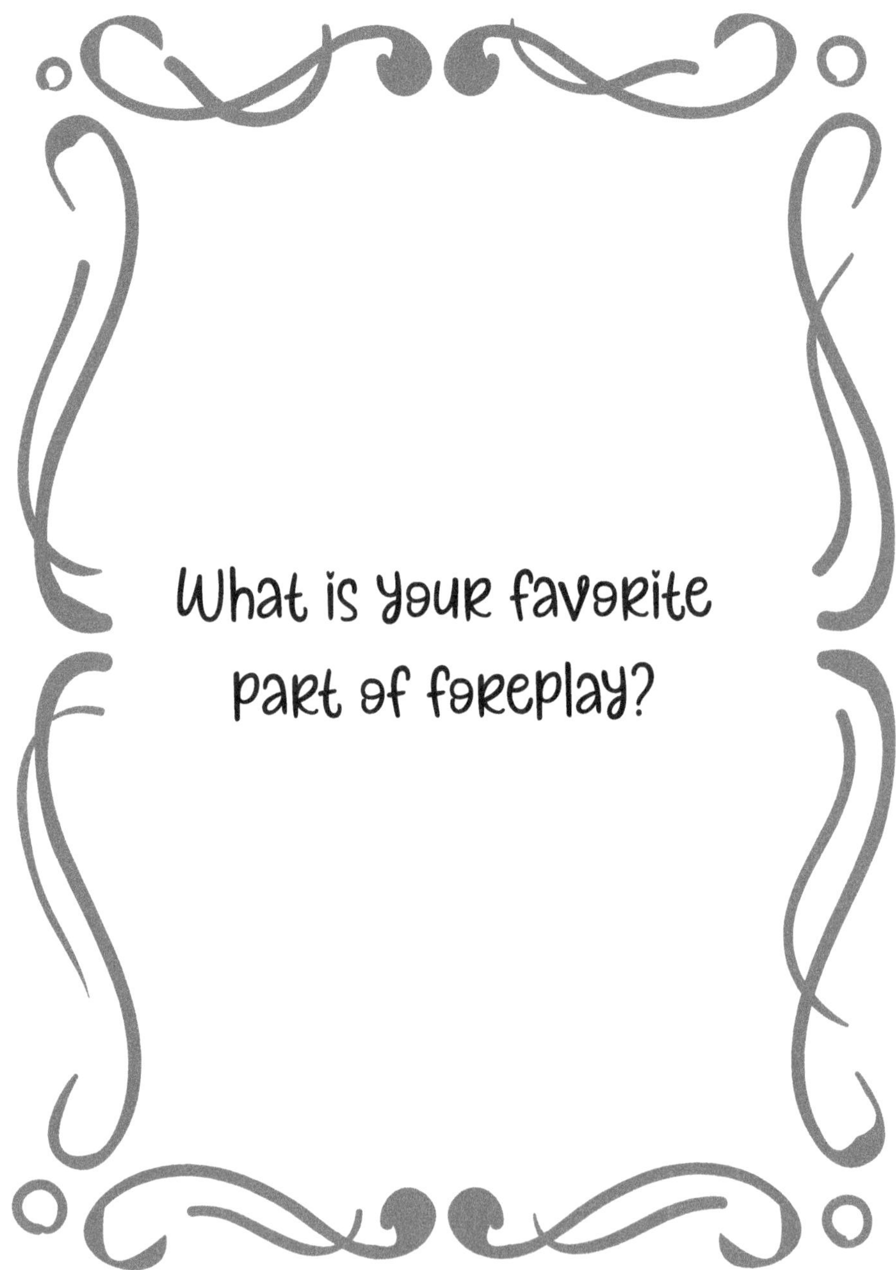

What is your favorite
part of foreplay?

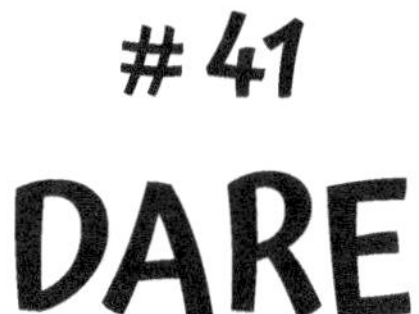

41
DARE

Whisper in my ear
something sexy about
me you've fantasized
about while you've made
yourself cum.

42
TRUTH

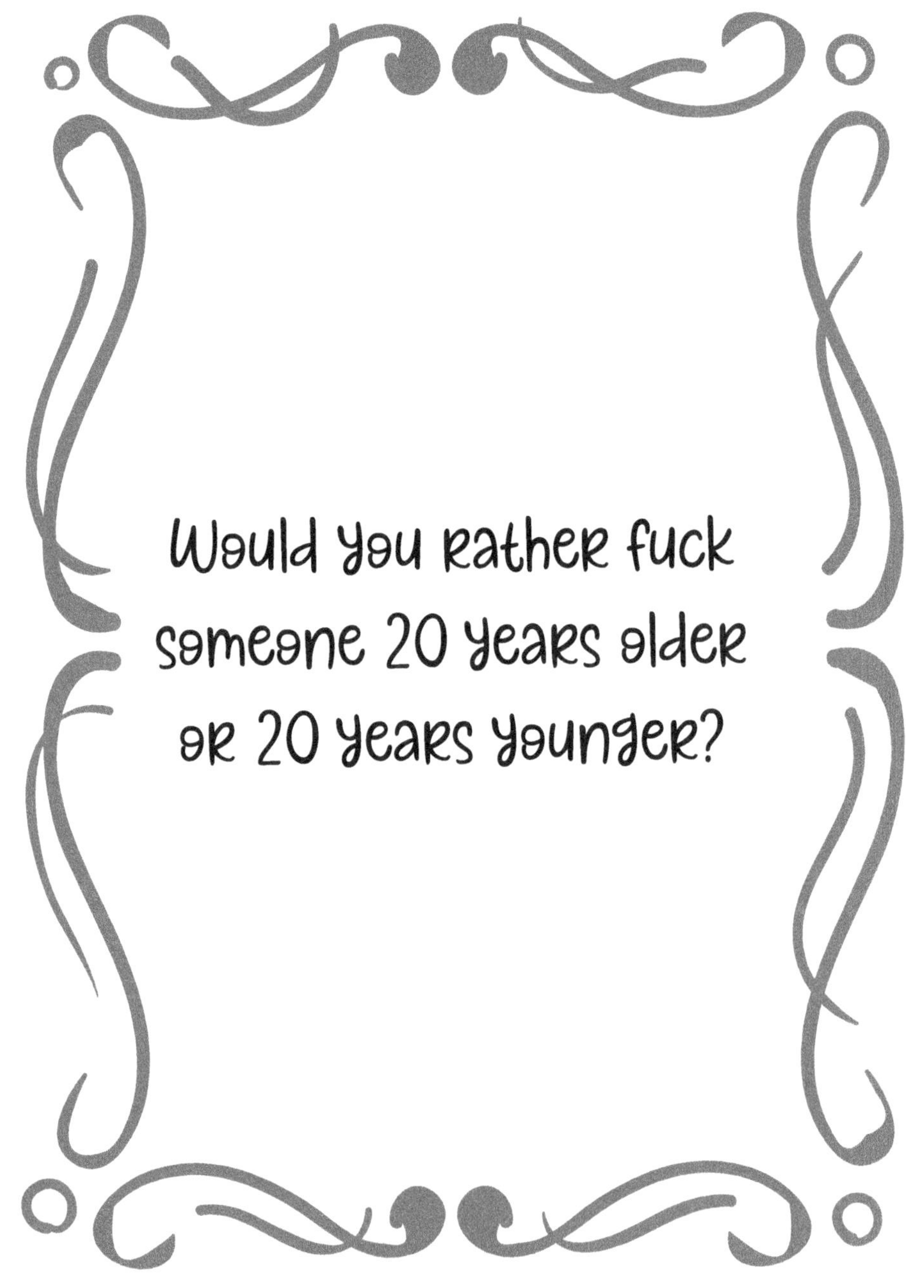

Would you rather fuck
someone 20 years older
or 20 years younger?

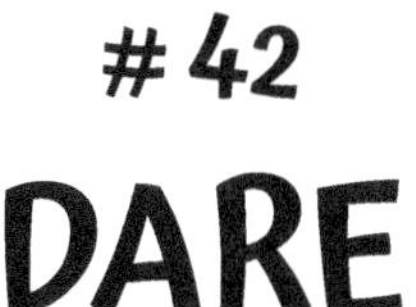

42
DARE

Kiss and lick my lips and try to get me to lose control and kiss you.

43
TRUTH

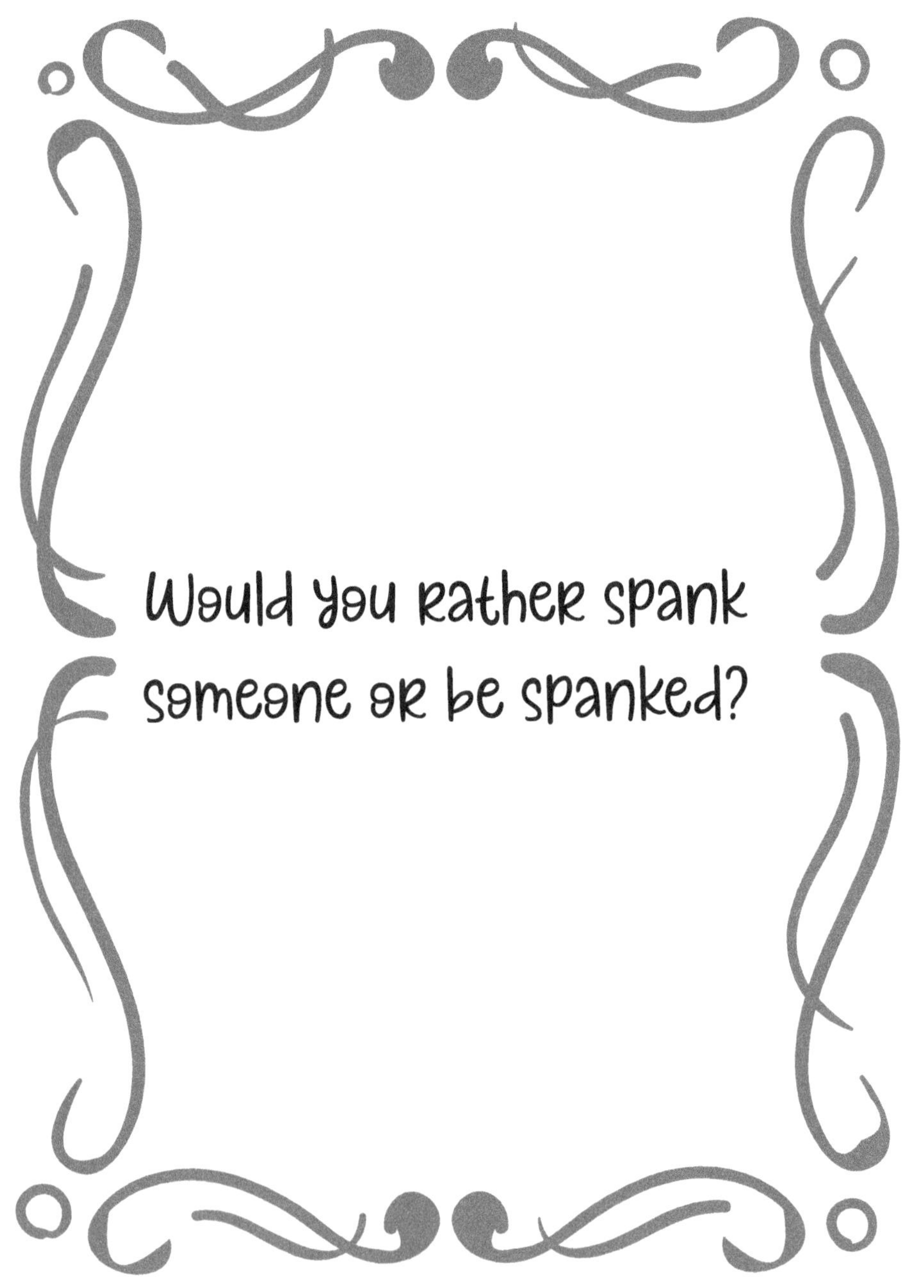

43
DARE

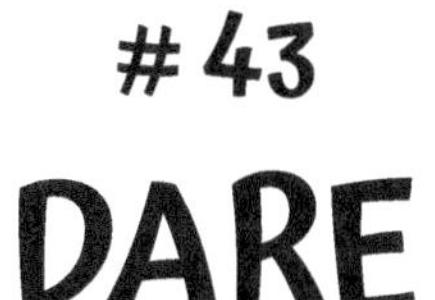

Show me the dirtiest image you have on your phone.

DARE

44

TRUTH

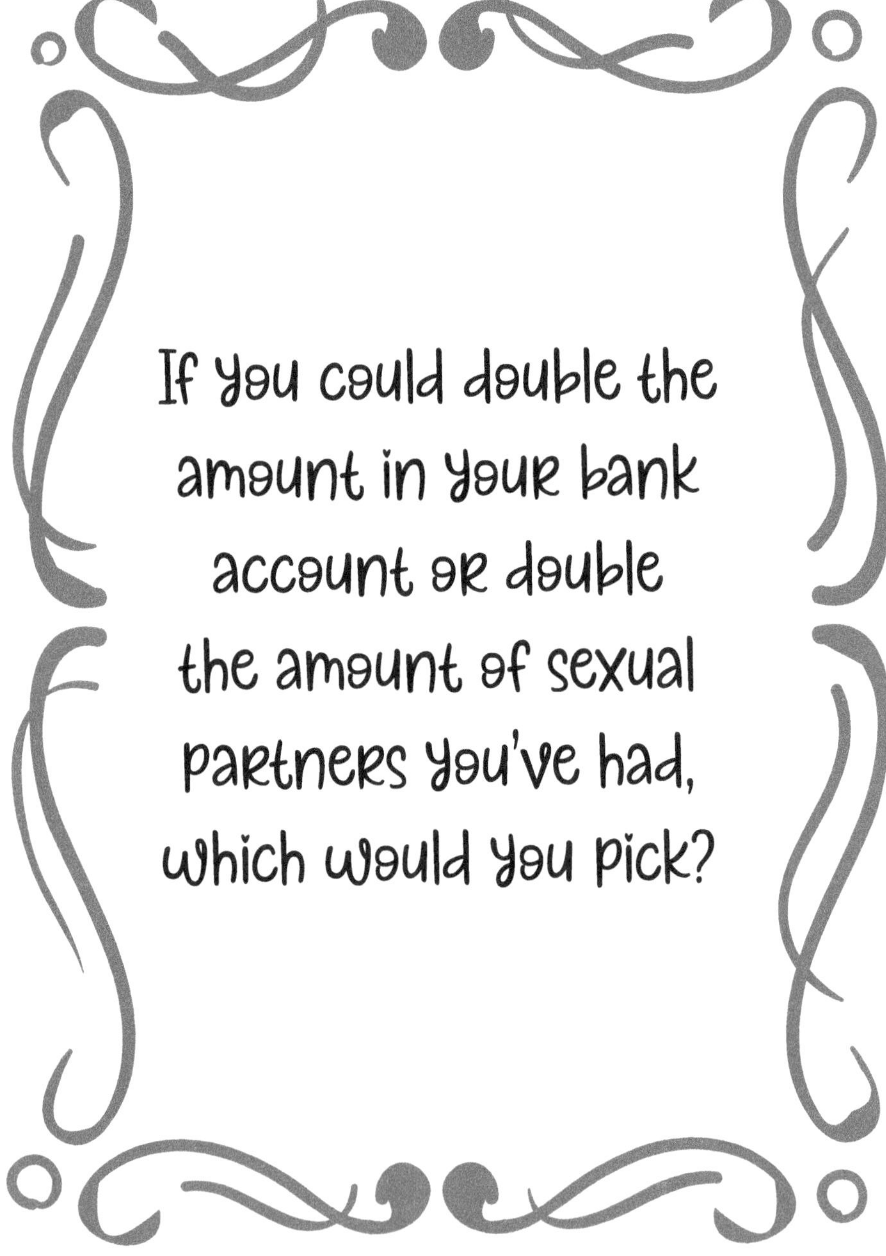

If you could double the amount in your bank account or double the amount of sexual partners you've had, which would you pick?

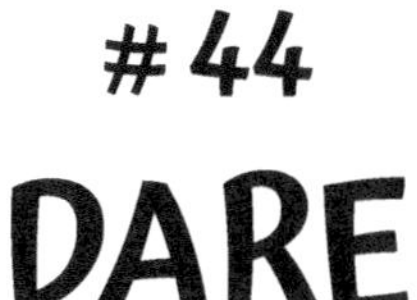

DARE

Pick up any book or
magazine in the room
and read from it as
seductively as possible.

45
TRUTH

Would you rather sleep with only insanely hot people or sleep with only people who think you're insanely hot?

#45
DARE

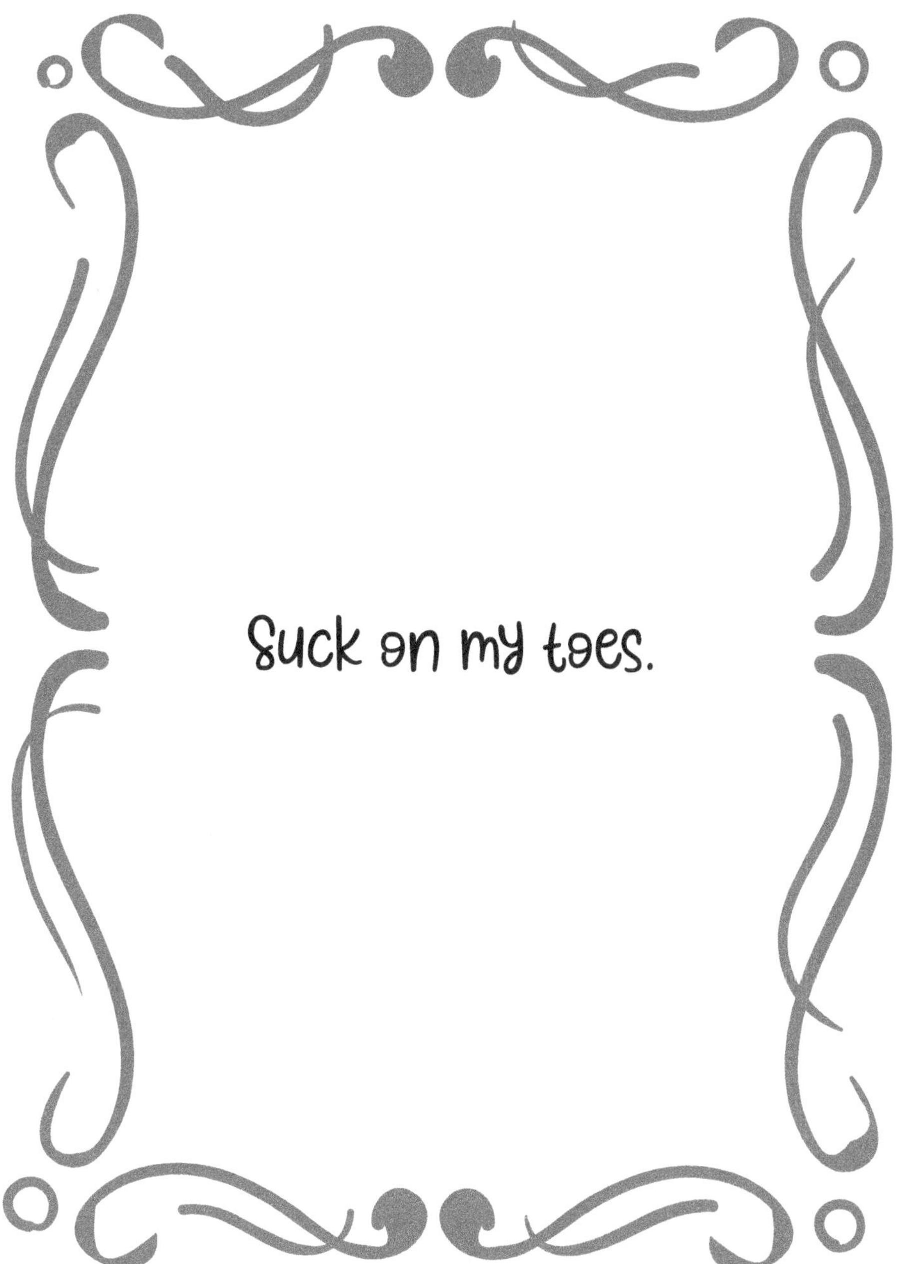

46
TRUTH

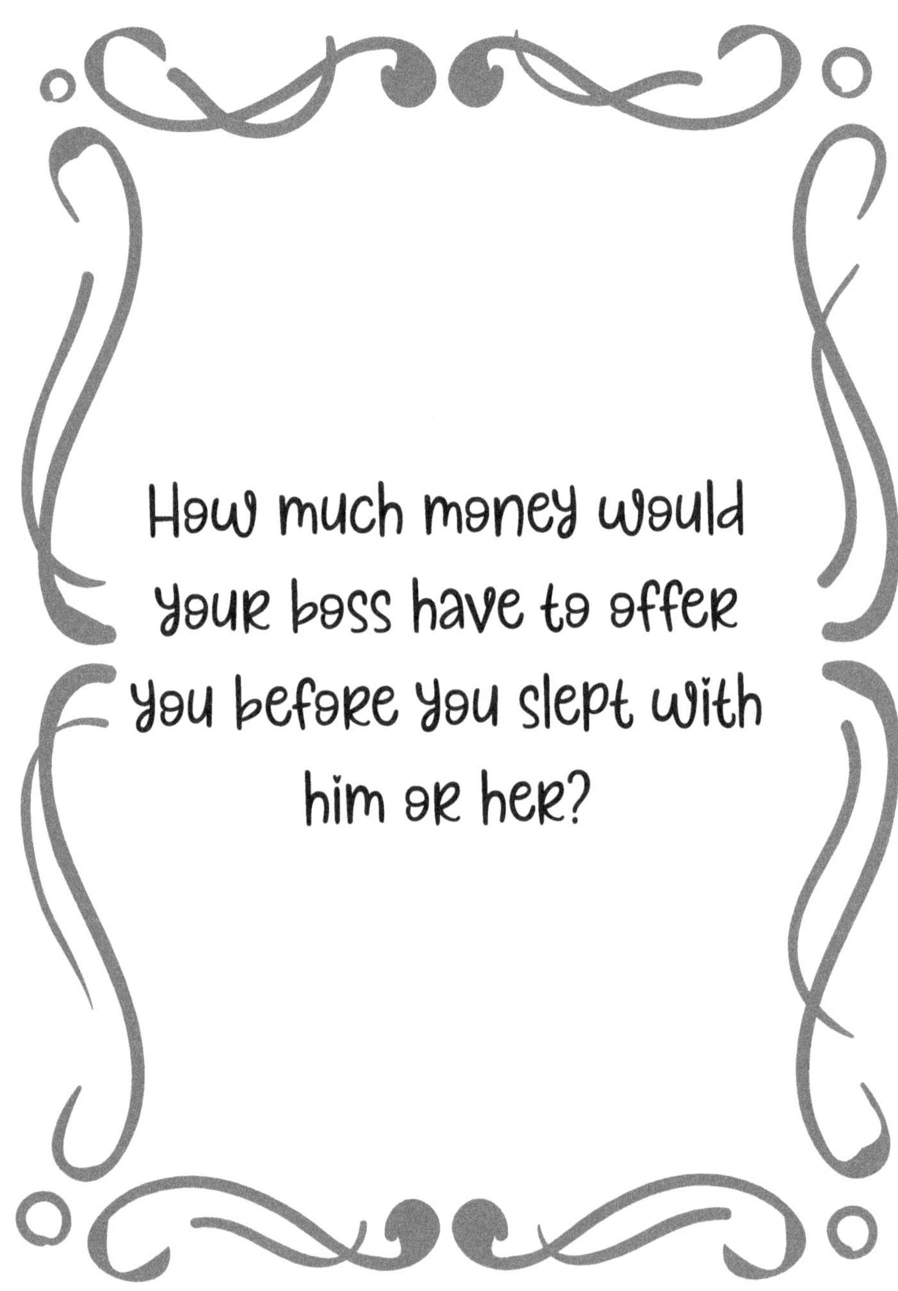

How much money would
your boss have to offer
you before you slept with
him or her?

DARE

Handcuff me and do something you've always wanted to do to my body.

47
TRUTH

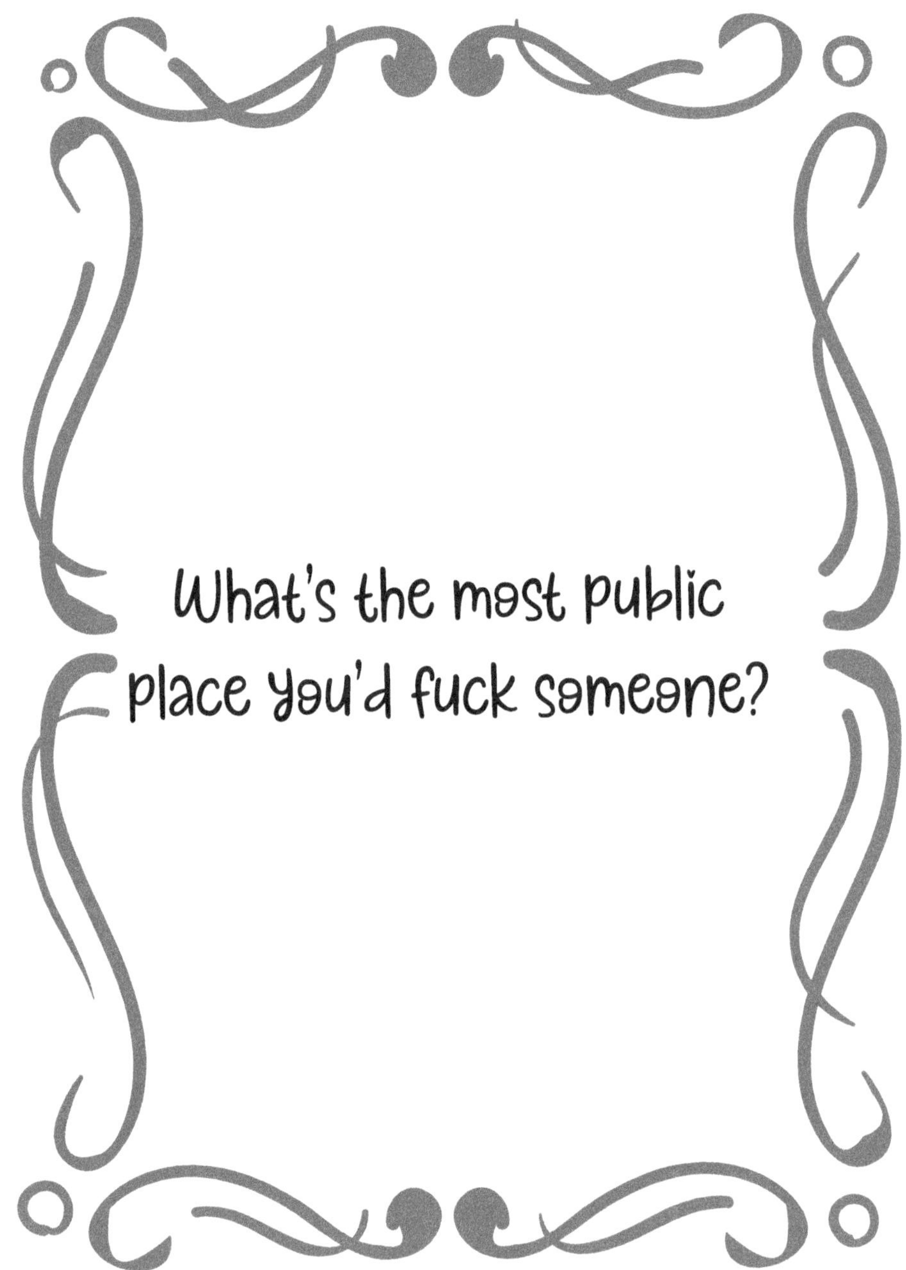

What's the most public
place you'd fuck someone?

#47
DARE

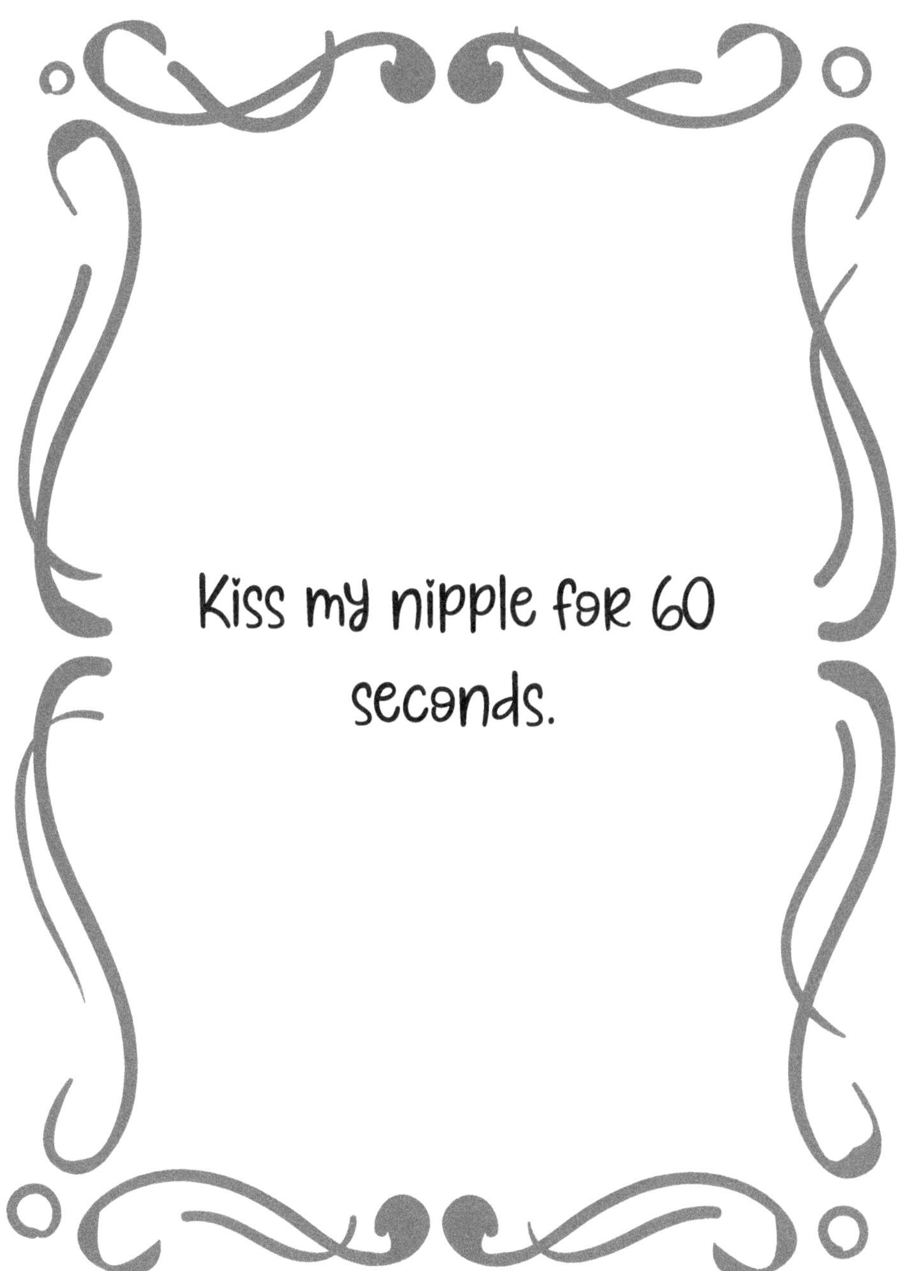

TRUTH

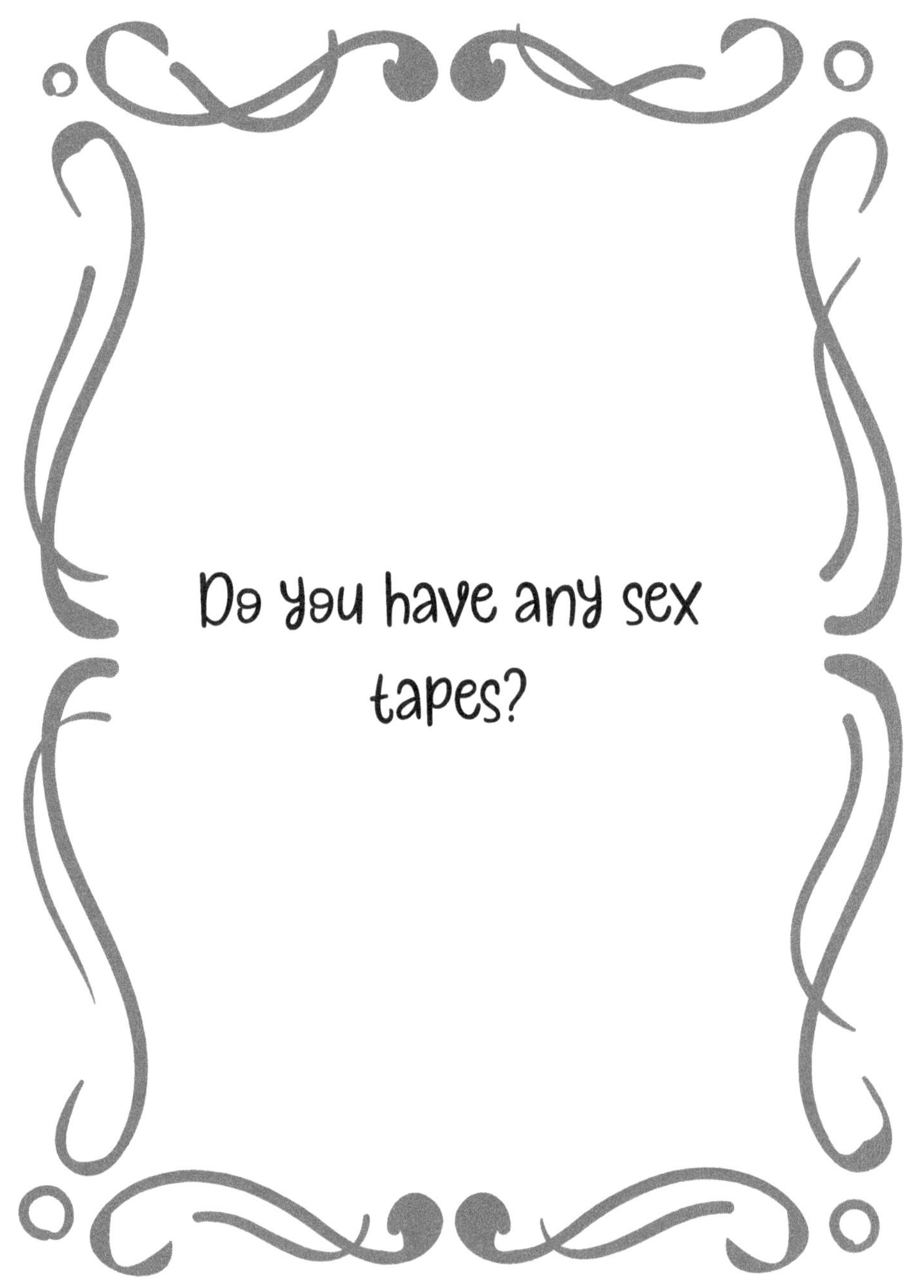

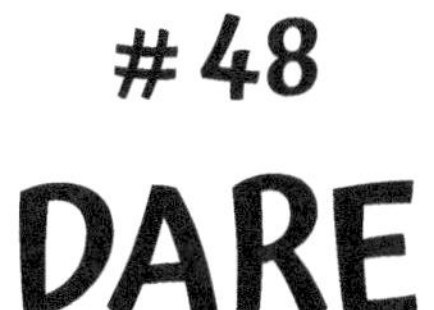

DARE

Try not to get turned on while I sit on your lap and kiss your earlobe for 60 seconds.

#49
TRUTH

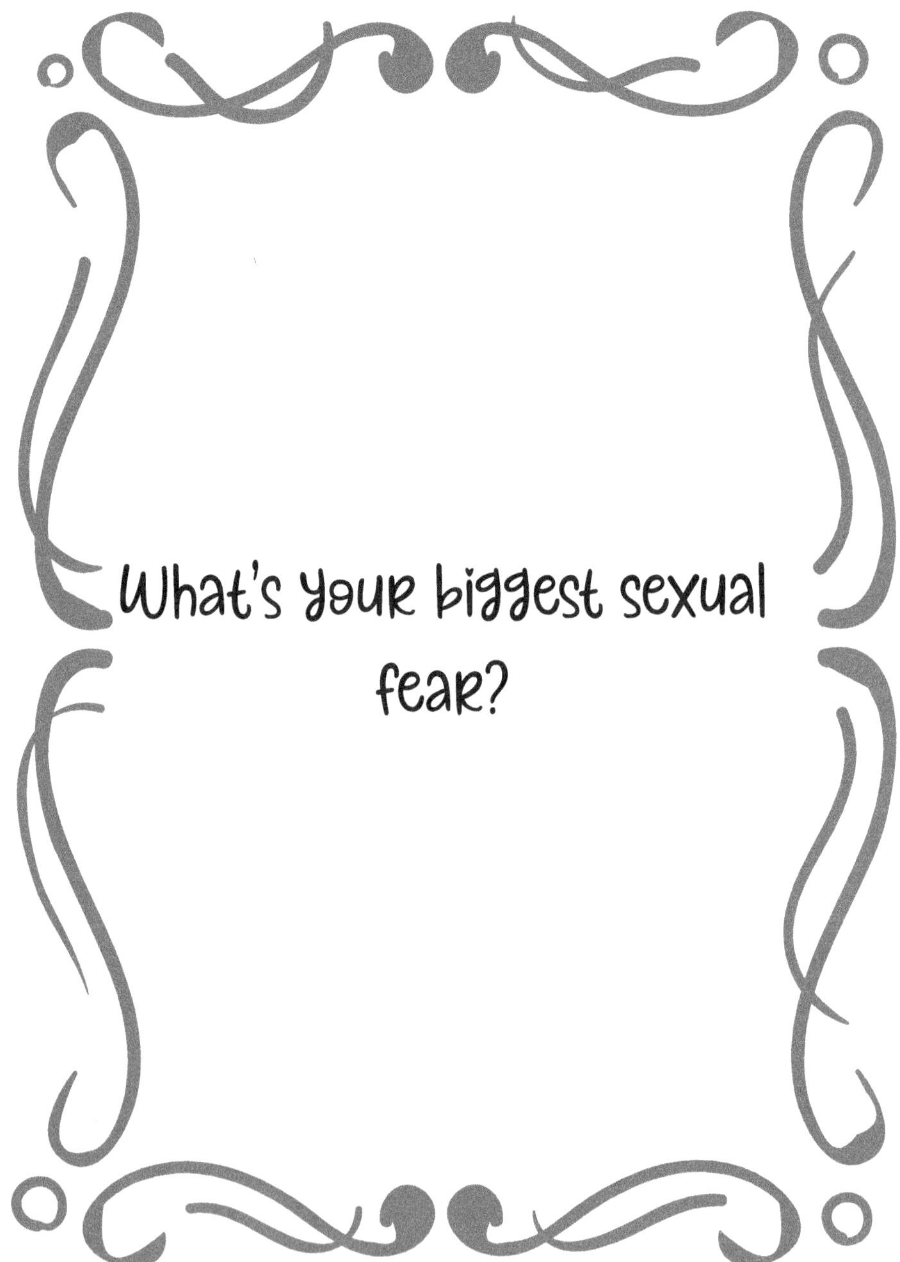

49
DARE

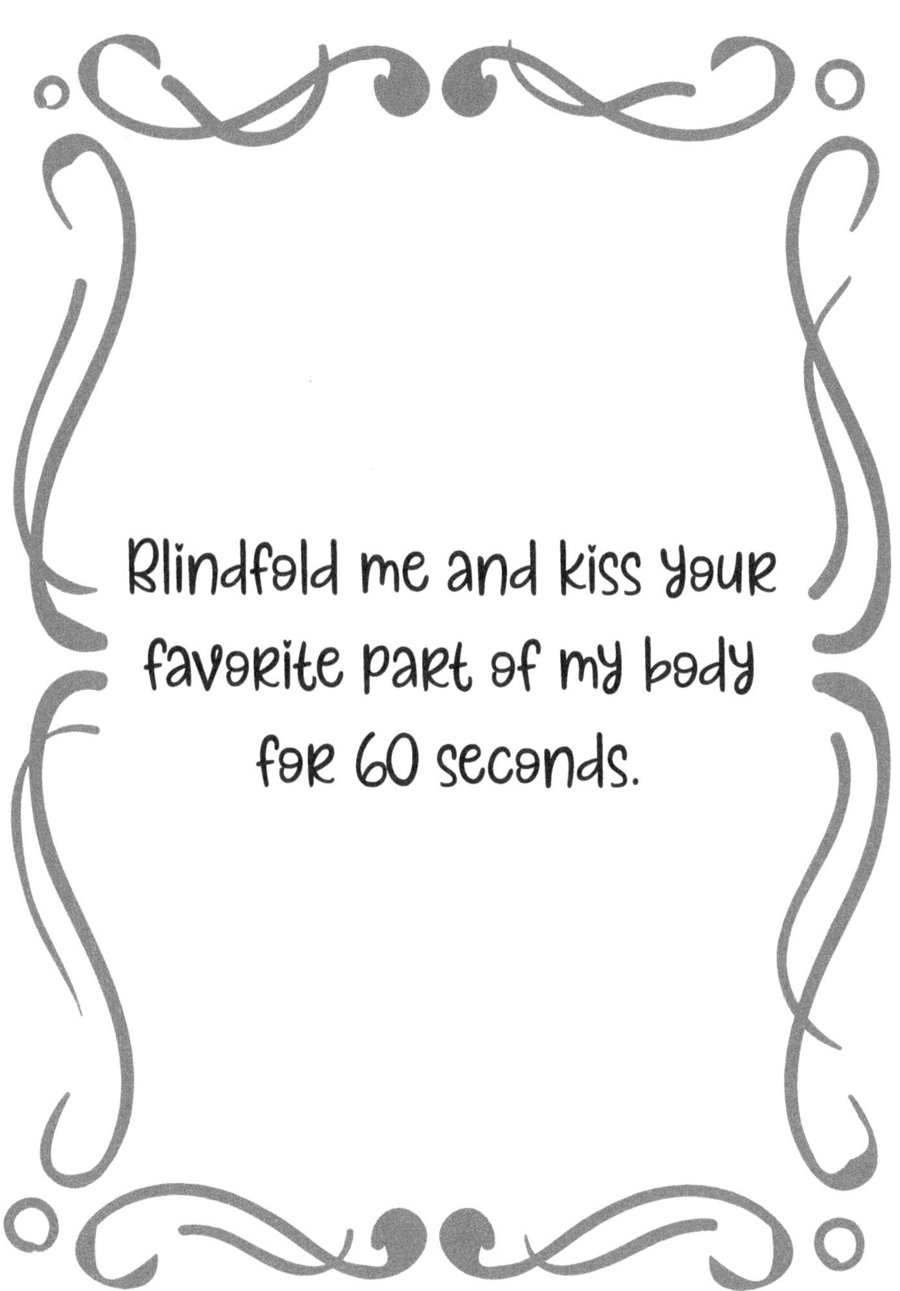

Blindfold me and kiss your
favorite part of my body
for 60 seconds.

#50
TRUTH

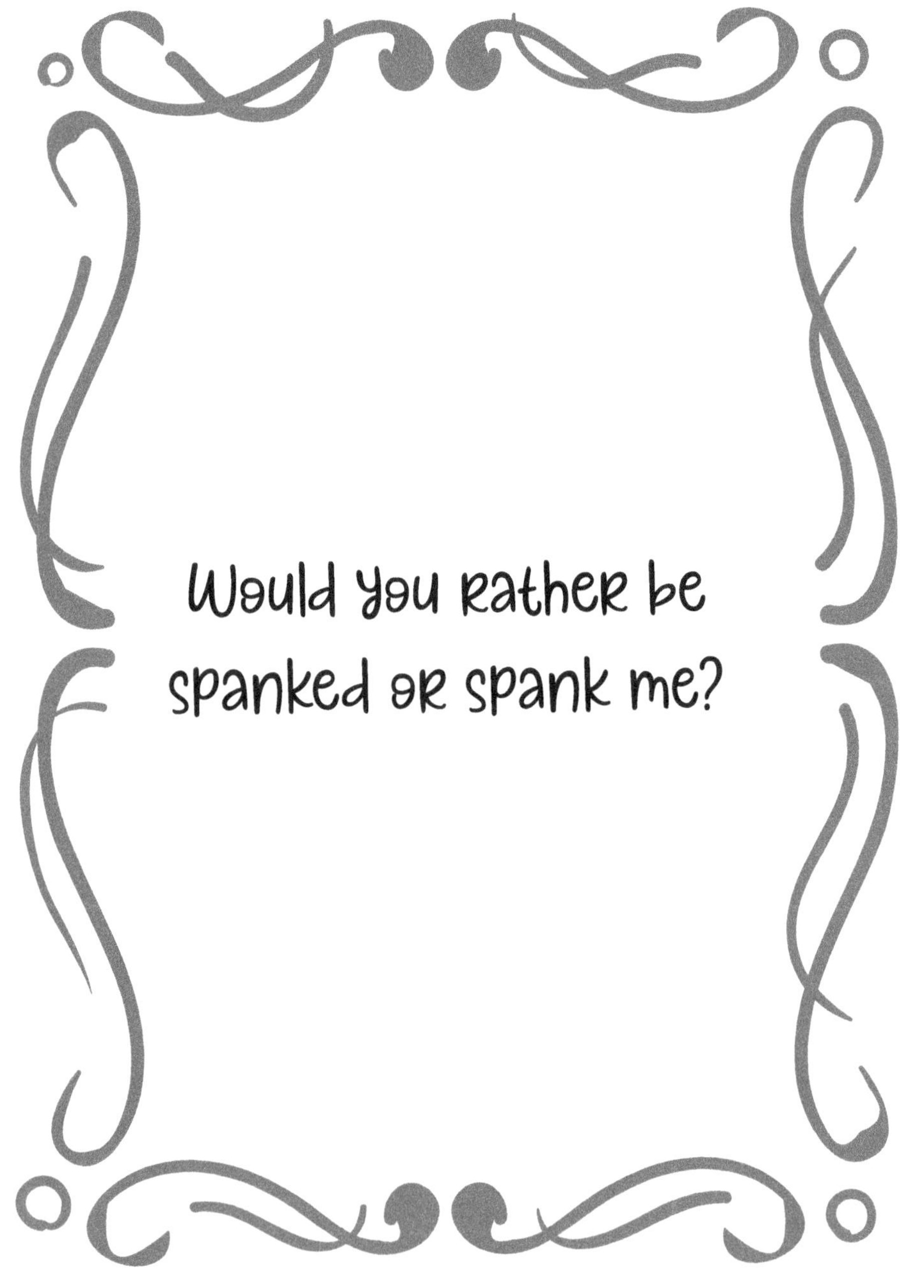

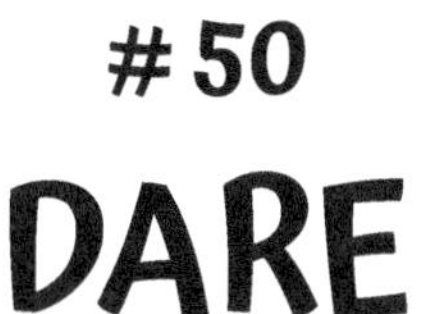

Send me the dirtiest text
you can think of.